The Gym Junkie's Guide to poetry

Your ultimate guide to fitness and health!

by Linda Skerman

illustrated by Owen Morgan

The Gym Junkie's Guide to Poetry
Text Copyright © 2017 Linda Skerman
Illustrations © 2017 Owen Morgan
Office images p61 - 68, stars p74 - 78, images p49 - 54 123rf

Published by Lilly Pilly Publishing, 2017
lillypillypublishing@outlook.com

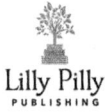

ISBN: 978-06481348-0-0 (print book)

All Rights Reserved. No part of this publication may be reproduced, stored in, or introduced into a retrieval system, or transmitted, in any form, or by any means (electronic, mechanical, photocopying, recording or otherwise) without the prior written permission of the author.
lindaskerman.author@gmail.com
Cataloging-in-Publication data is available at the
National Library of Australia

Dedication

This book is dedicated to my Trainer, Tom Crocket; to my Kinesiologist, Doreen Logan and to the leaders of the Max, International College for Fitness Professionals, Kman, Rowie and Steve.

I would also like to thank my husband, John, my daughter Jo, my friend Lyn and the lovely ladies and gents at Toowoomba Daytime Squash for their support and love.

Thank you all for your immense support in helping lift me from the quagmire and into the light.

This book is also dedicated to those in search of answers. I hope this book can simplify the mystery around health and fitness, giving clarity and direction to your own fitness journey.

May you all be healthy, fit and strong for life! - LS

Contents

Imagine i

PART ONE: *The Nuts and Bolts of a Happy Bod!*

So Much Information 2
I Don't Have Time to Be Healthy! 3
Compound Exercises 5
The Trainer's Perspective 7
The Program 8
Super Compensation 9
Too Many Push-Ups 10
Recovery 11
Spot Reduction Exercises 13
Too Many Sit-Ups 15
Fitness Fads 17
The Secret 22
Professionalism 25
Squash Poems – The Bad Sport 28
Fifty 30

PART TWO: *All About the Food*

The Diet Wheel 32
The Never Ending Diet Roller Coaster 35
What To Eat 36
Beware - The Lucrative World of Impression 37
A Little Anatomy and Physiology 38
A Case of Intimidation 42

PART THREE: *The Art of Being an Entrepreneur*

Les Mills- International Glory 44
A Chat with Zig Ziggler 49
The Amazing Walt Disney 55
Why Do Businesses Fail? 61
The Risk 70
Who Am I? 72

IMAGINE ...

Imagine if a sit up
Could give you abs of steel
But you forgot to do your legs
You'd end up like an eel!
Imagine if your arms
Could triple in their size
But you forgot to do your butt
How would they ever rise?
Imagine if your legs
Were powered like a gunner
And all the fat fell off your arms
What would you do this summer?
I've got a funny picture
Computer generated
Of bits of us we made just right
And others that were fated
No fat upon our face
And too much on our ankle
Now that would just be all too much
And get us in a rankle
We'd have to get it right
Use labs and much precision
Take a bit and add to there
Let's use a deep incision
I think it's gone too far
This lack of common sense
Let's take a look and see what else
Could work without offence ...

Part One...

The Nuts & Bolts of a Happy Bod!

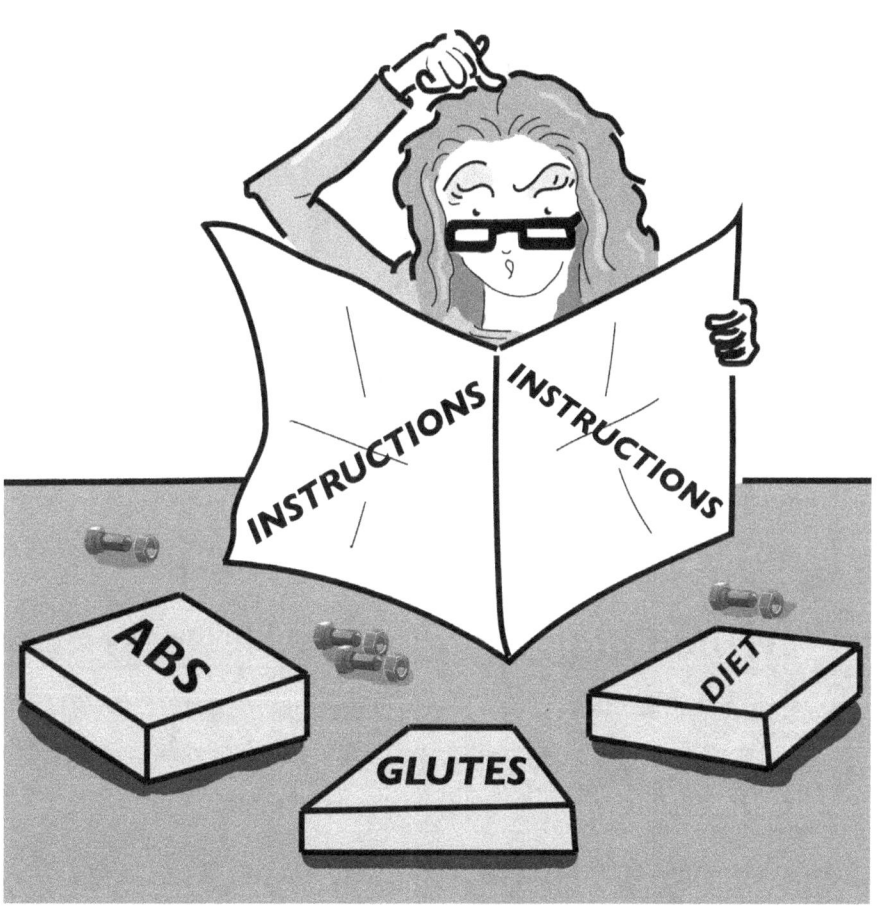

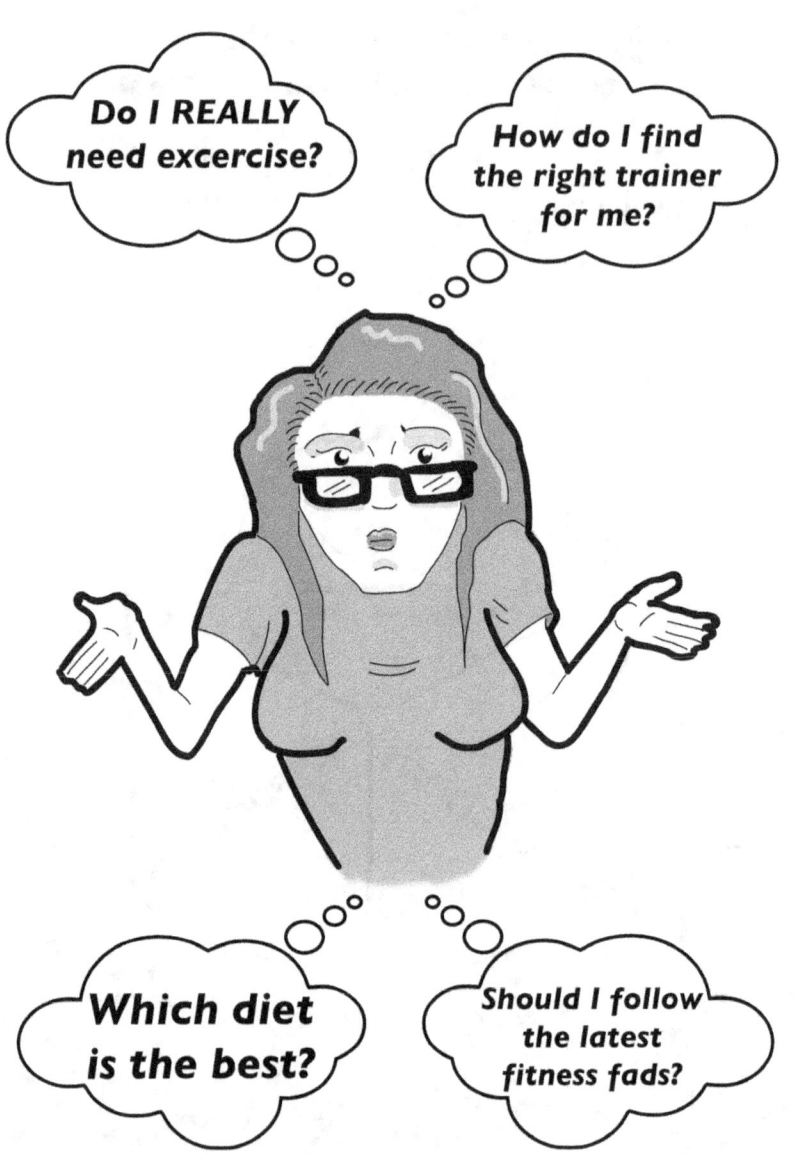

But... I Don't Have Time to Be Healthy!

I don't have time to be healthy!
I don't have time to be fit!
I don't have time for all that hype
I won't buy into it!

All the money in the world
Won't get me to that gym
Mr Universe is not my fan
I won't end up like him!

I see the fads, I see the fans
I see the money pit
All those people in the mirror
Looking, oh, so fit

I see the room and all the weights
Those great big bars and things
It scares me off just seeing that
They all are ding-a-lings!

Too many mirrors and I'm so fat
How could I walk in there?
I see the people in my mind
And all they do is stare

Little kids with all that muscle
What do they need it for?
What's that got to do with me?
I find it such a bore

I know I'm fat but aren't we all?
I am just like all the rest
I think of fit and I give up
I'll never pass that test

I should go out and take a run
I should do stuff, I know
I want a better look and feel
I want that healthy glow

continued...

So many thoughts, so many fads
So much to gather in
Where to find the stuff for me
Where do I begin?

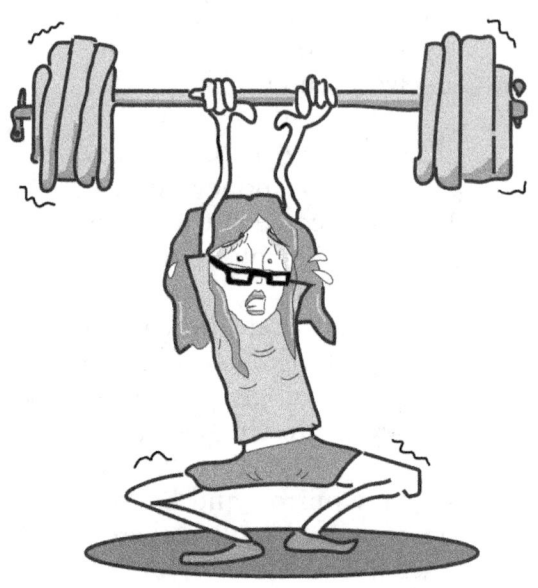

Compound Exercises ...

Compound exercises replicate function
Not just cutting off a joint at a junction
Would you like to run, hop, skip and play?
Doing such activities each and every day?

Copy off the movement you would do in life
Don't just do a 'bicep curl' and get yourself in strife
Great big movements for a great big life!
Looking quite fantastic for your husband or your wife!

When you train 'big' the hormones release
Giving you results as you would see your strength increase
Lifting 'heavy stuff', of course it is all relative
Will give you markers you can see, it can be quite comparative

Using lots of muscles improving your joint action
Not a thousand sit ups that would bring about impaction
Joint stability, this function is so needed
Not much fun to lift your arm and find it is impeded

Train your whole body, keep the power strong
When you lose the weakest link, you will not last for long
You want to be a champion! You want to be a star!
Don't overtrain the weakest link, for you will not go far

Could you count the muscles you're doing in a squat
I guarantee that you will find that there is quite a lot
The big ones that we know of, the hamstrings and the quads
But what about the rest of you that's holding up your 'bod'?

Give your 'bod' a challenge, back and front and sides
When doing squats you'll find there's so much more goes on inside
I couldn't count those muscles, I couldn't count them all
All I know is one day they could stop you from a fall

Another thing I'd like to say is 'Why train on the floor?'
When you're in an upright stance, you can do a lot more
In doesn't make much sense when you are on your back
Is life for you one great big bed on which you are a stack? *continued...*

So train yourself while standing, that's where you live your days
Forget about the crunch and see, there are much better ways
Do your crunch each morning when you get up to play
Just one of them will soon suffice to get you on your way

And have a lovely life, be healthy, fit and strong
Live your life up with the gods, it is where you belong
Enjoying every moment, because you are the star
I hope that life is good for you, I hope that you go far!

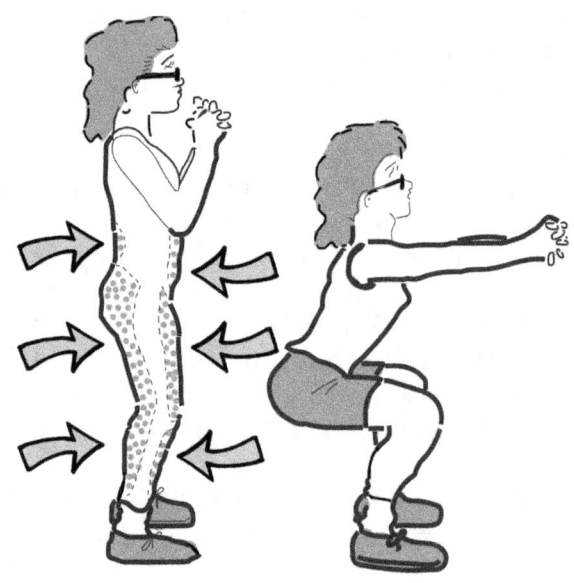

The Trainer's Perspective ...

When you get a client
Who walks into your door
Don't sell them all the hype'n stuff
That's not what they're here for

Keep it short and simple
Remembering their goal
They want to love and laugh at life
They want to have control

They need a simple answer
They need your common sense
They do not want a task too great
They do not want a fence

They need to see a vision
An answer oh, so sweet
They need a goal that they can reach,
A target they can meet

So teach them 'huffy puffy'
Teach them to be strong
Help them with their food a bit
And then you can't go wrong

For time is of the essence
It's everybody's blame
It is the reason they hold back
They're punting on that game

So make a little gamble
That's what you're here for
Keep it short and simple, love
And they'll come back for more!

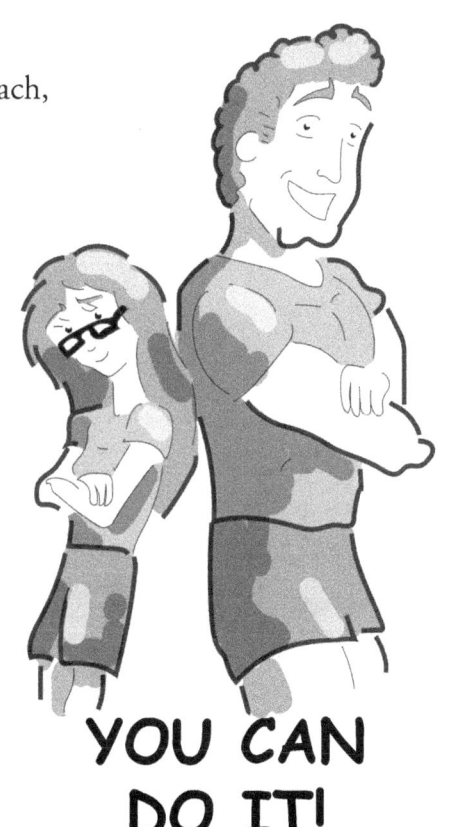

YOU CAN
DO IT!

The Program ...

When you make a program
Of course you will decide
That squats and push ups are the best
Don't take them on some ride

You'll find a starting measure
A weight that's fairly easy
Ask them how they want to train
Please, don't let them get queasy

You'll take them to their limit
Whichever one they choose
Remind them what it is they want
Their goals and visions use

And when their session's over
Make sure they take a break
For when they rest and eat some food
Good gains then they will make

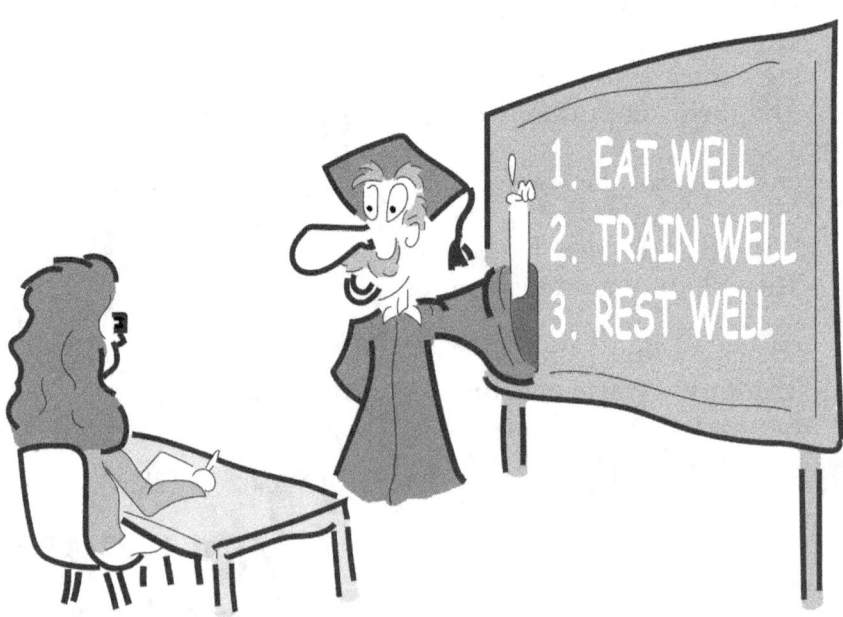

Supercompensation ...

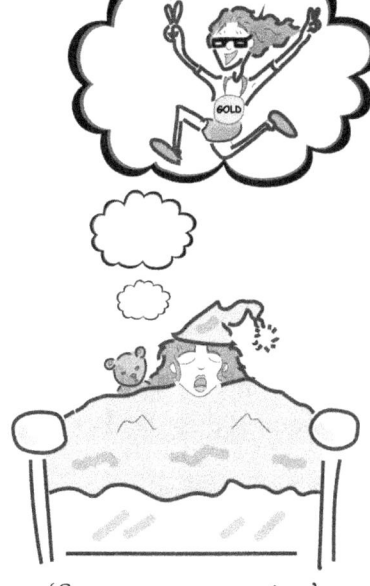

'Supercompensation'
A term that's new to me
Is what the body does with rest
It does it perfectly

When you train your body
As hard as you can do
It does a little damage
To cells and muscles too

The nervous and hormonal
These systems in the body
Are slightly shocked and need a rest
Or they will get quite shoddy

There's quite a lot of work
That goes into improvement
Who would think that all this comes
When we involve some movement?

The body needs a moment
In which it will recover
Your gains are made in rest, my friend
It's what you will discover!

Too Many Push-Ups!

Or the Science of Overtraining ...

Too many push ups won't make a man
You need to make it as hard as you can
Pushed to your limit, now you will feel
Something so tangible, something so real

Fatigue and a tiredness, you're in distress
Go home and take a bath, you need a rest
Decline in performance, no more can you do
For if you don't rest these things will ensue ...

All of your body is feeling so drained
Most of your muscles and joints are in pain
You might get sick a lot more than norm
Watch for your ligaments they might get torn!

You might feel restless and grumpy at stuff
Does this sound bad and have you had enough?
Losing your leanness, some fat creeping on
Lacking some sleep? This does not look like fun!

Worst of all things from an athletic view
Failure to finish what you want to do
Regression, how sad, now you're getting weaker
All because you were a gym pleasure seeker!

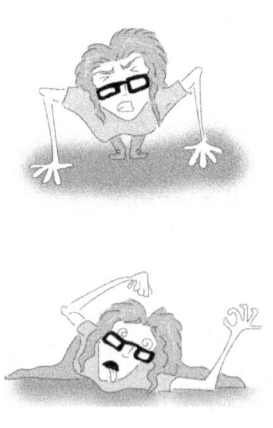
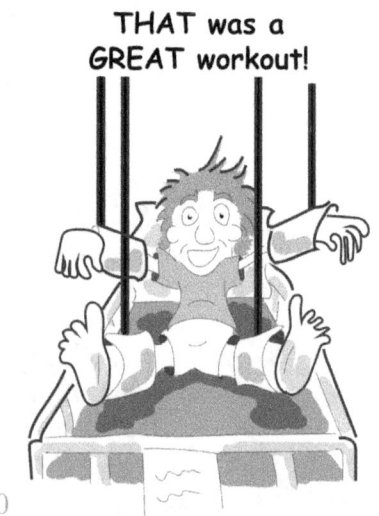

RECOVERY ...

How <u>do</u> my muscles get stronger?

Protein synthesis
Your body is rebuilding
All the little bits of you
That need a little gilding
Taken to the limit
Now you can be stronger
Next time you can lift some more
Or go a little longer

The particles in muscle
Like fibres in a rope
Have broken down a little bit
And now they cannot cope
They need to lay more fibrils
They need to have repair
The myocin and actin,
Now need a little care

Like workers on a house
When walls have seen some damage
We need to build it stronger
So that next time we can manage
Your body is amazing
It always wants improvement
That's why you need food and rest
To make a better movement

It will not settle back
One moment on its lees
Not settling for second best
It always tries to please
So if you want to be
A stronger person quicker
Wait until the body makes
Your myofibrils thicker!

continued...

I'm waffling, I know
But science is amazing
And when you get to understand
You may do some rephrasing
Your training will be clever
No wasting of your energy
Keeping up with all your plans
Aligning, using synergy

So there you have it, friend
I hope you will be wise
When training hard to make a change
I hope you get first prize!

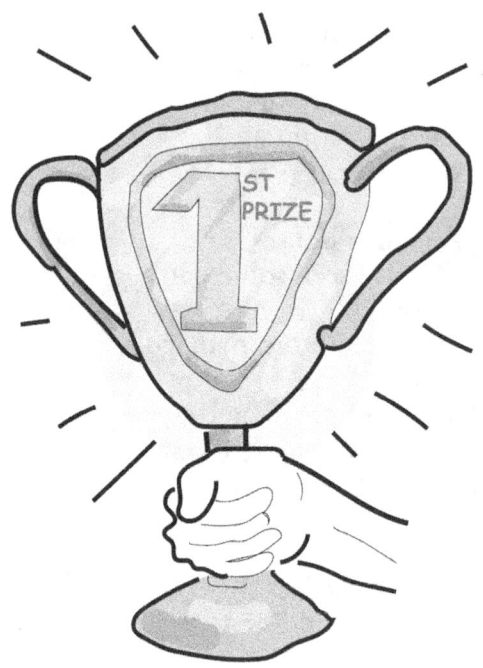

Spot Reduction Exercises
Do they really work?

How much fat does a crunch burn off?
How much muscle does it make?
How many days till I see my abs?
How much time will it take?

How many 'bicycles' must I do
Before I lose my 'tyre'?
How much time can I hold my plank
Before I feel the fire?

How many times must I 'sit-up'
Before I lose my urge?
How many of these wonderful things
Will it take my fat to purge?

I want that look, the fashion pic
The perfect tone and tan
I want to be acceptable
To each and every man

I'm so focussed about my core
I want my fat to go
For then I can go to the beach
And put myself on show

My fitness mag is such a help
I hear the writers say
"Follow our great plan to get
Your thousand sit-ups each day"

The 'latest research' on the news
The latest toning app
Will help me get my legs in shape
So they don't look like crap!

continued...

I'm so serious about my goal
I'll follow any fad
I'll find some 'awesome' training plan
So I don't feel so bad!

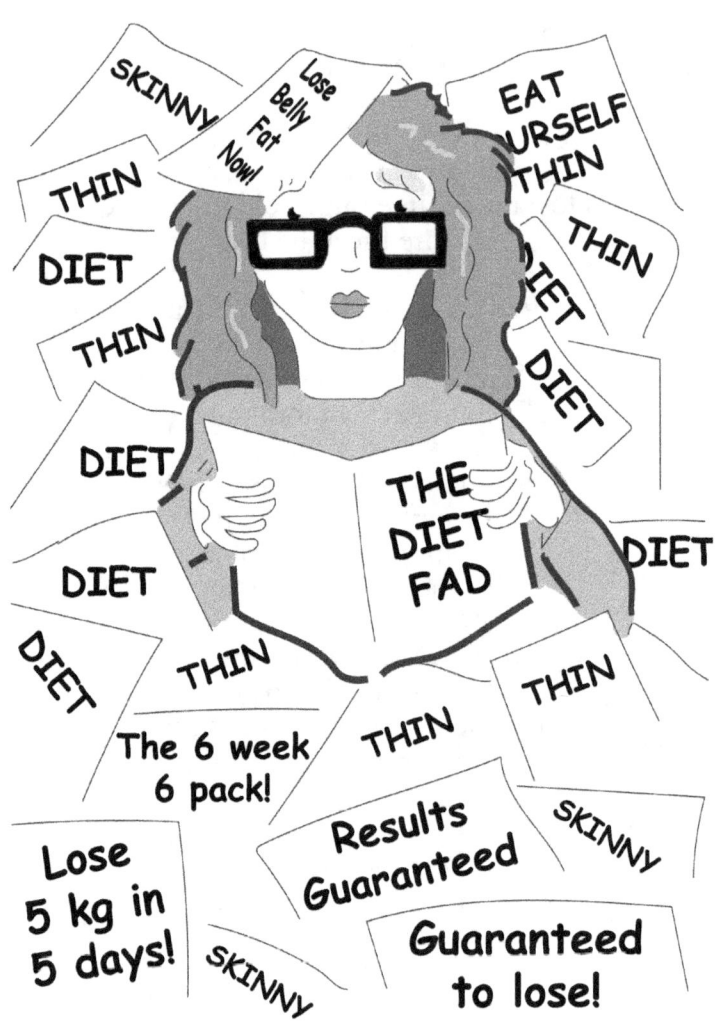

Too Many Sit Ups ...

Or what happens when you follow a fad ...

I once had a spine that worked in conjunction
With all of my muscles, aligning, with function
I'd walk and I'd run and life was a dream
I had that young glow, I had self esteem

I was a perfectionist all must be great
Until one sad day I found it my fate
That I could not walk without pain in my back
Because of the way how my spine did not stack

Sorry to say but this fact I divulge
That too many sit ups had caused a big bulge
That when from the thousandth sit up I was getting
I found such a grief and my spine was now letting

Not holding me strong like it did before
I found that I could not get up off the floor
The damage was bad, could not be undone
The pain that I felt, it was really no fun

'Herniation', a terrible word
Is something I know, it is rather absurd
It's something that happens when you follow a fad
Intelligent man is quite often so sad . . .

The insight of years would now like me to say
Don't follow that path there's a much better way
Instead of believing that you'll fix a 'spot'
Don't fall for that fallacy, go for the lot

It's so hard to fix a spot here or there
And if you would try you will end in despair
The body's and organ complete and entire
And you must regard it a little bit higher

continued...

Don't go for the quick fix, use your insight
Training yourself will take more than one night
Use movements that replicate all of your day
For that is the answer, that is the way

And then when your body is getting much stronger
You'll probably find that you'll live for much longer
When thinking of exercise, think as a whole
Something that's good for your heart, mind and soul.

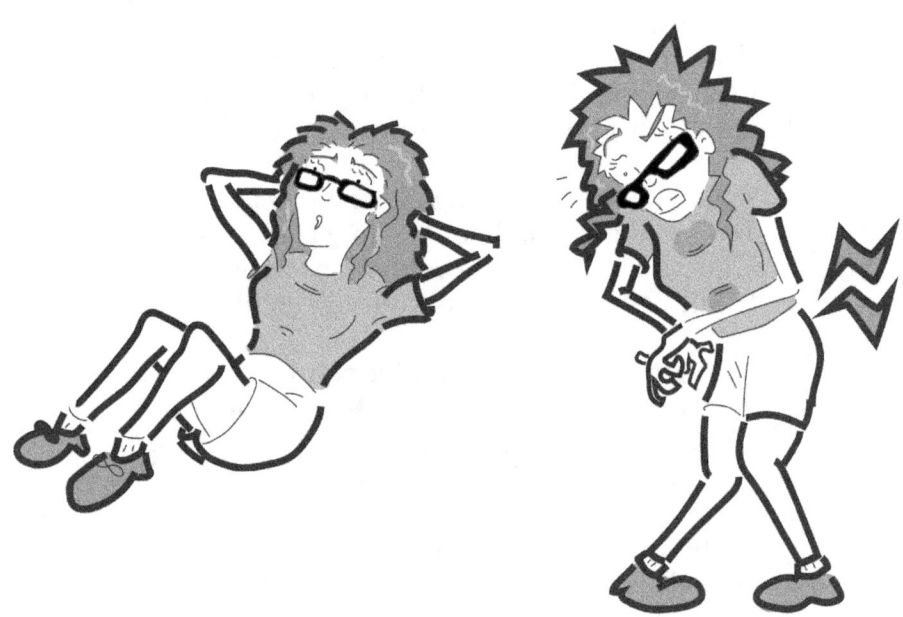

Fitness Fads ...

If you want a body
That's health fit and strong
You may need to readjust
Your sense of right and wrong

For you see there's many fads
Will lead you all astray
Showing you a lot of stuff
That's causing much delay

Look into a mirror
Don't be nonchalant
Take a moment and consider
What it is you want

Fit enough to take a run
Strong enough to play
Healthy bones to lift you up
And power through your day

Lean and quite good looking
Muscles we can see
Energy for living life
And much vitality

What you want is splendid
It is quite universal
But how and where you take advice
Can be quite controversial

continued...

There are many views
So much philosophy
Some of them are just plain daft
And some like comedy

Some will tell you plainly
To follow their example
But what they have to offer you
I would not want to sample

I have heard of many fads
I will name a few
'Rollerfit' and 'Retrosweat'
'Dragonboating' too

Hang on now, I think there's more
You could be on air
Yoga moves done upside-down
Pilates on a stair

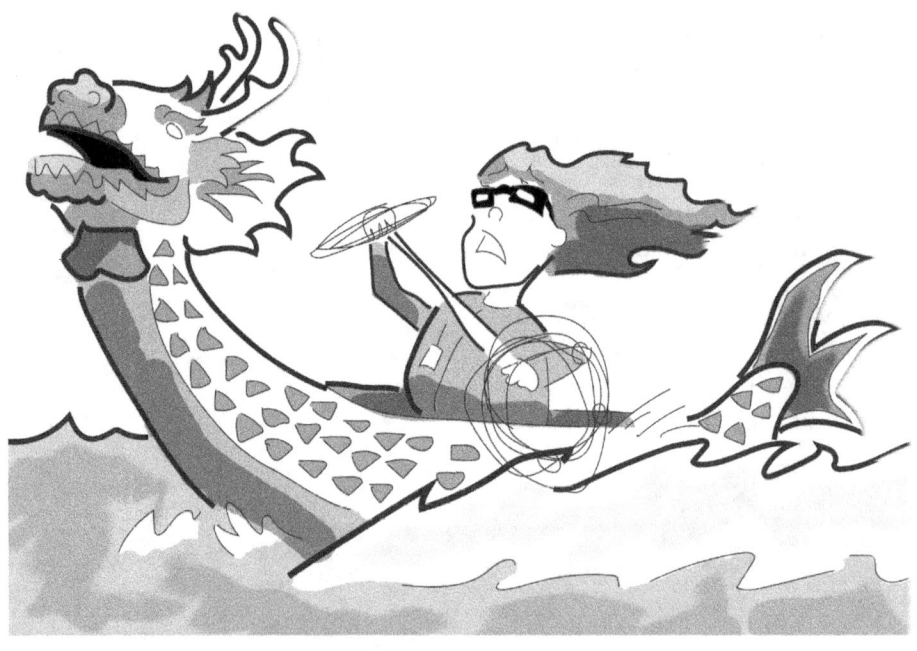

Now some of these are funny
And some are just plain dumb
And honestly you may be better
Off, if you did none

What we need is something
That makes our muscles work
Not just flitting here and there
And following some quirk

What we may not see
Is that we are a body
And when we overuse our joints
They will become quite shoddy

Decline will come quite quickly
With all that wear and tear
And soon you will discover that
You have no padding there!

Anti-Gravity Yoga
Hanging from the ceiling
Sounds like a lot of fun
But will I be a stronger version
Of me, when I'm done?

Will it serve my purpose?
See me through my life?
Or will my health decline with age
And I end up in strife?

Can I do the shopping?
Carry all my bags?
When I am still tied up
To the ceiling in some rags

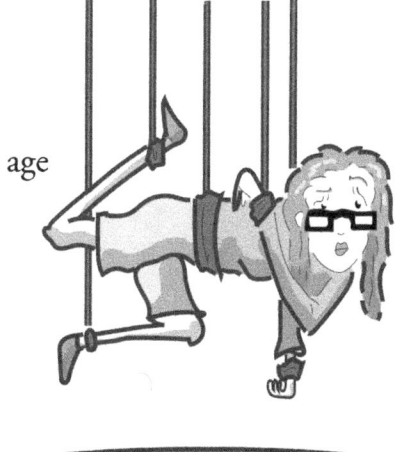

Can I lift the grandkids?
Walk around the block?
Does my body cope and
Does it know which way is up?

continued...

Crossfit
Doing lots of chin-ups
So many in a row
Is something else that can be used
To put yourself on show

Meeting with some others
The workouts are repetitive
Put them all together in a way
That is competitive

What we may not see
Is that we are a body
And when we overuse our joints
They will become quite shoddy

Decline will come quite quickly
With all that wear and tear
And soon you will discover that
You have no padding there!

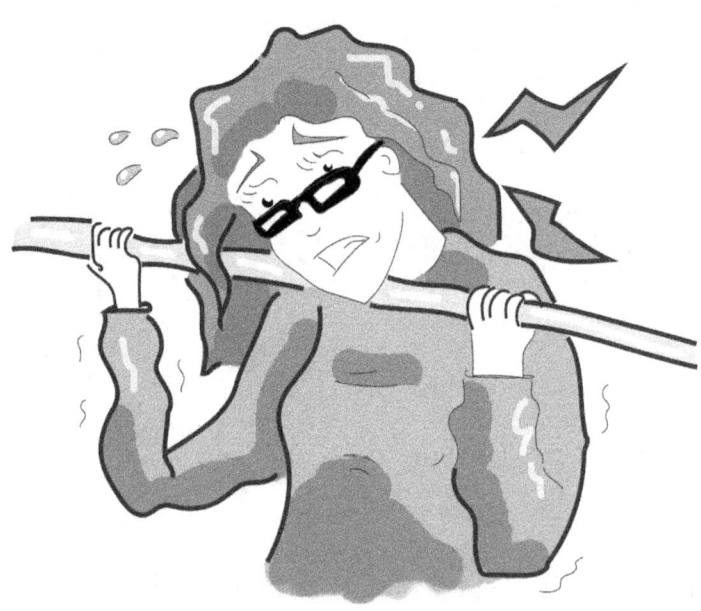

Retrosweat
'Retrosweat', a workout
Something from the past
If you like the eighties
You might find it quite a blast

Doing all those grapevines
Dancing like Jane Fonda
But will it make your muscles strong
I cannot help but wonder

Yep, sure, it looked quite fun
Remembering the stuff
But if you find you're short of time
It just won't be enough

Lifting heavy things
Was nowhere in the set
You'd think we'd learn by now
It's like a game we call roulette

Rollerfit
I could try a class where I do
Exercise on skates
Apparently it's quite a lot of fun
With all your mates, but

Lifting dumbbells while on wheels
Sounds something like a farce
And all I have is visions of me
Falling on my 'arse'

THE SECRET?

Find yourself a trainer
Who has his head on straight
And get yourself a program now
Before it is too late
Make sure he is clever
Knows how the body works
Keeps the program simple and
Without those other perks

Lift some heavy things
Don't do it very often
Once a week may just suffice
Don't end up in a coffin
Make the choice right now
It's with your life you're dealing
Something you can stick to and
That you will find appealing

When you're lifting heavy
These things you should approve
Functionality, using
All your compound moves
Thing like squats and deadlifts
Push ups and the bench press
Lat pull down and chin ups
Are the ones that will impress

Using your whole body
Makes perfect sense to me
If fact it is much more aligned
With your reality
Keep it short and simple
Don't complicate the wheel
Then when you are eighty
How magnificent you'll feel

Your joints will be well oiled
And you will feel a treat
Your bones will be as strong as steel,
And you will shun defeat
You'll breeze through life so steady,
'Cause you preserved yourself,
And you will have a body
That's a picture of good health

In summary I add
When you would think of motion
Just look at how a man is made
Forget all this commotion
He lifts a pile of wood
Is running from a bear
He climbs into a tree to find
Some food for his own fare

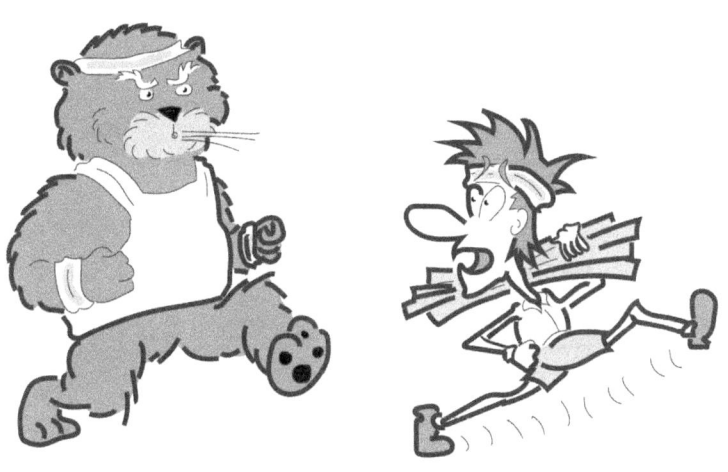

These actions are our basics
The way we all are made
To make our bodies fit and strong
These rules must be obeyed
So make a plan and you will get
Results that you desire
Do not follow superficial fads
From which you'll tire

If you stick to basics
Results are guaranteed
Don't just follow any crowd
Don't follow that stampede
Be bold and stand alone
If that is what you must
Find a mentor who has sense
One that you can trust

Find yourself embracing
The courage from within
Committing to a goal you want
A vision you can win
Own your own best body
Be constant every hour
You will feel invincible
And you will feel the power.

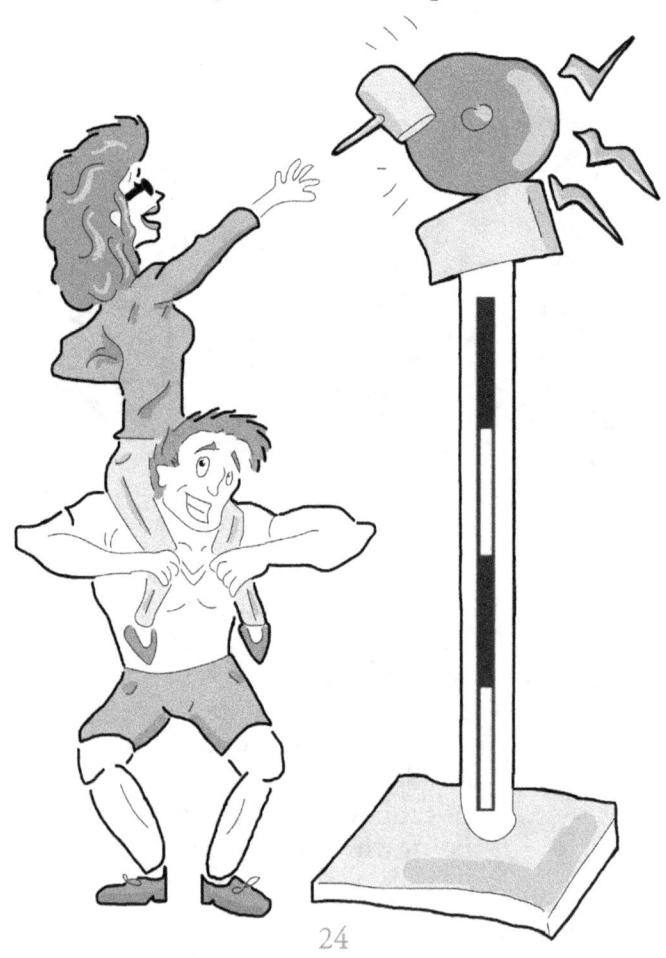

PROFESSIONALISM

OR the art of finding an Amazing Trainer!

Look smart
Please be neat
Have some good shoes
On your feet
Collared shirt
Tuck it in
Don't wear too much
Of that bling

Tailored look
Don't be slack
Please don't show me
Your six pack
I need people
I can trust
Good example
Is a must

Bright eyed
Bushy tailed
Make sure my time
Is emailed
At the door
You'll be waiting
There to meet me
No debating

Big smile
Warm greeting
Open questions
When we're meeting
Ask a question
About me
Treat me like
Royalty

Who am I?
What's my mission?
What's my plan?
What's my vision?
What's my drive?
Motivation?
Do I have
Determination?

To achieve
My desires
Do I have
What it requires?
I need help
From this profession
I rely
On your discretion

Please be awesome
Look a treat
If you don't
I might retreat
Be on time
Be prepared
Inside I am
Really scared

Make me feel
Quite at ease
Melt my heart
Don't let it freeze
I need help
From a person
Don't let me
Decline or worsen

continued...

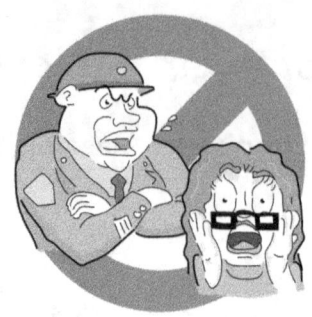

Like a doctor
Or a nurse
Help my troubles
To reverse
Your profession
Is important
Have the look,
The deportment

Know your value
You save lives
You're an angel
In disguise
Help me focus
Show me moves
Gain some strength
My health improves

I need health
For my life
So I don't get
Into strife
Know your value
To the nation
Saving lives
Your occupation

Your profession
Number one
For the good times
And the fun
See your value
Be the light
So we don't
Give up the fight

Learn the reason
Know your stuff
Or I might see
Past your bluff
You could help me
If you're willing
Your example
Is instilling

Let the world
Know your name
Prevention is
A better game
Keep us all
Strong and healthy
Inside we are
Very wealthy

Your profession
Health and fitness
Your example
Is a witness
Keep it simple
Do it right
Stand for something
Be a light

When I speak
Of your name
I will spread
Abroad your fame
Cause you are
Like a friend
One on whom
I can depend!

"My assignment
You will see
How I act
Professionally
Highest standards
I declare
Showing people
That I care."

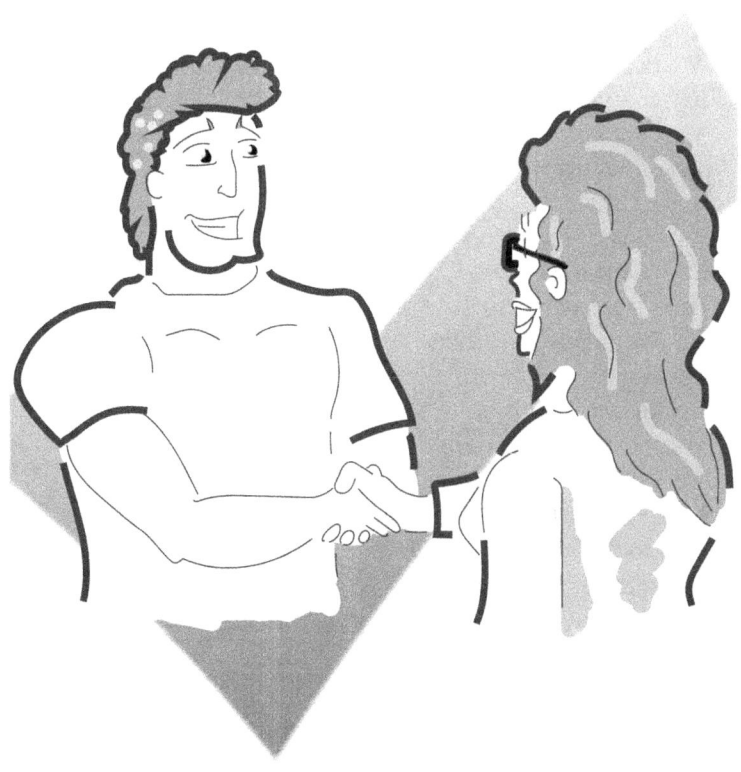

A Little Squash Ditty!

The Bad Sport

The player crowds
Crashes
Condemns
And curses!
He spits accusations at the umpire!
And demands
Attention
He wants to win!
No matter the cost!
For loss
Means a dint
In his ego
He doesn't know
What it means
To be a good sport
On the court
He is a bully
He pushes
And wrangles
And strangles
The air of warmth
He is cold in manner
And hot
Under the collar
And if you paid me a dollar
For every curse
And every complaint
And every display
Of lack of constraint
I would have my
Squash fees paid
For the next year
Or maybe two!
So next time you
Go on the court
Don't be caught
Into thinking

You're with friends. . .
It just all depends
On the luggage
They bring with them
You must be prepared
For anything
Laugh or cry
Pain can sting
But you can sing
Your song
Be strong
And 'don't take no crap'
From any ill-timed
Mishap
Or bad tempered person
Whose state will just worsen
As soon as you start winning!
From the beginning
Let them know
You're not here for show
But to give it
Your best go
And to play fair
And to have fun
And when you
Go on the court
I hope you get the good sort
The one that is
That good sport!
And always remember
To be one yourself
For that, my friend
Is your wealth!

Fifty

Fifty straight drives up the wall
Fifty drop shots with that ball
Fifty boasts and that's not all
Fifty lobs, now watch them fall
Fifty volleys from the back
Fifty more now use some tact
Fifty cross-courts, watch me run
Fifty more, now aint this fun?
Fifty drills to keep me fit
Fifty more to use my wit
Fifty drives that keep to length
Fifty backhands, see that strength!
Fifty serves, I'm almost there
Fifty from the other square
Fifty times, I'm just beginning . . .
Ten thousand more,
And THEN I'm winning!

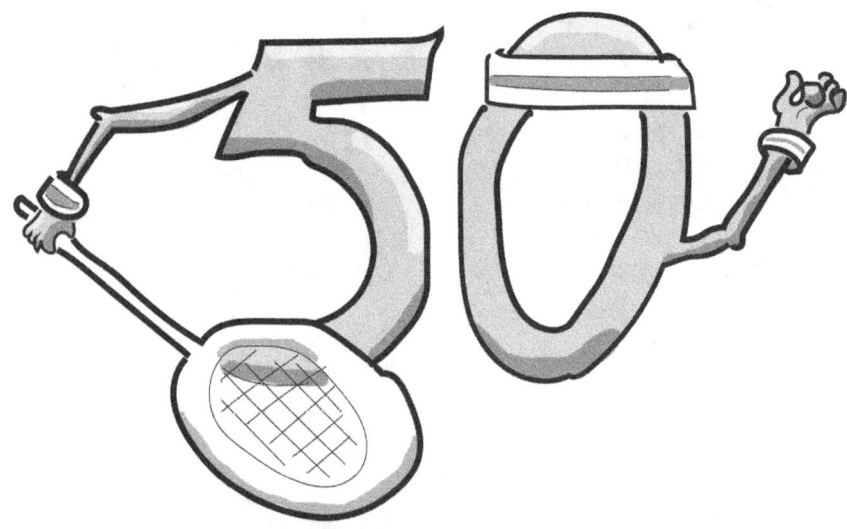

Part Two ...

All About the Food

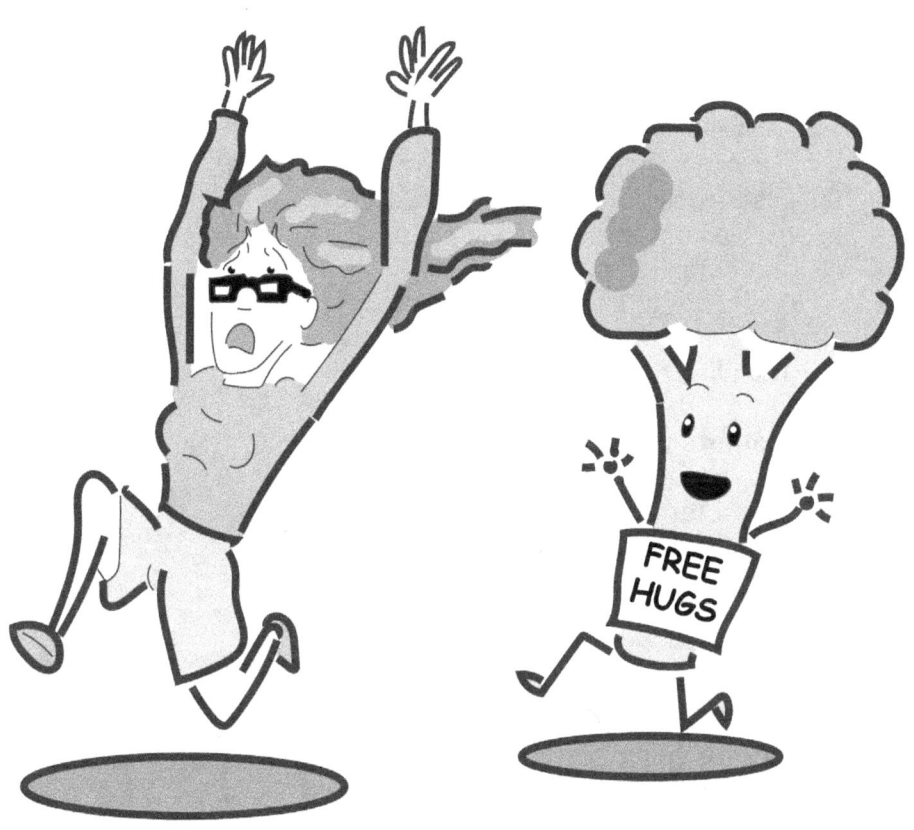

The Diet Wheel

The diet wheel goes round and round
Sometimes you are up, then you're down
Restriction just hurts
There are no sweet perks
To something else now you are bound

The moment that you want to do it
You see food and then want to chew it
The things that you love
Are the foods you can't have
And your meals end up tasting like suet

Desire
The body that seems so illusive
Leads to actions that are quite abusive
It's like a mirage
Some mixed up collage
Available to the exclusive

The gloss
On the diet you're choosing
Promises pounds to be losing
But the fad of the day
Could just lead you awry
And you'll find your life much more confusing

The 'Zone Diet'
The 'Zone Diet' by Doctor Sears
The 'wisdom' of man now appears
"Controls gene expression
Hormonal repression
And keeps you young all of your years"

The food that you eat must be measured
All 'junk' from your life should be severed
High protein a must
Most carbs you will thrust
And his book must be bought and be treasured

So if you like eating a 'sanga' (sandwich)
Or even your mash and a 'banga' (sausage)
You won't like this plan
From this 'well-informed' man
Whose mere words sound like one great big clanger

Now if you find all this a muddle
Don't worry, don't be in a fuddle
His products online
Will suit you just fine
Send money into his great puddle

The Blood Type Diet
So now we will take a brief look
At the "first and the only great book"
That gives "unique" advice
(And it's only half price!)
By our blood type our food we now cook

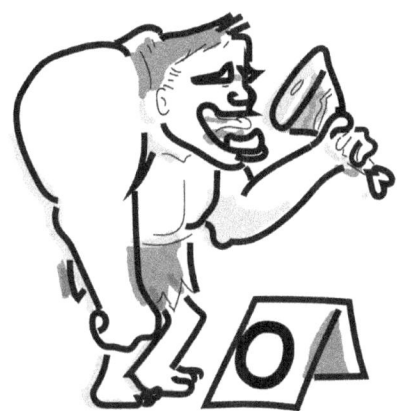

So if I am classed as an 'O'
To my ancestors now I must go
I should eat lots of meat
Almost nothing that's sweet
Like the caveman that lived long ago

Or if my blood type is an 'A'
The vegies are meat for today
I should do my yoga
While wearing my toga
Be calm and play golf in the day

continued...

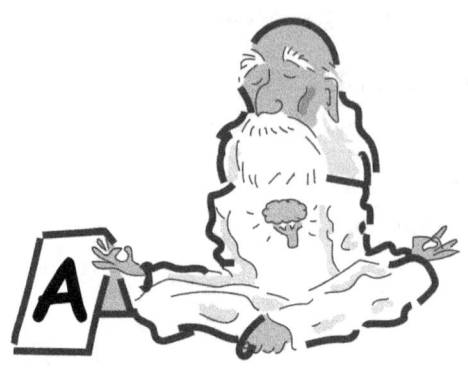

For those with a blood group of 'B'
Most foods you can eat, you're lucky
If you're one of these ten
You can eat where and when
Dr D'Adamo makes his decree

So is this all fiction or fact?
Is it all from the evidence backed?
I can tell you one thing
Your back pocket will sting
The science can't ever be tracked

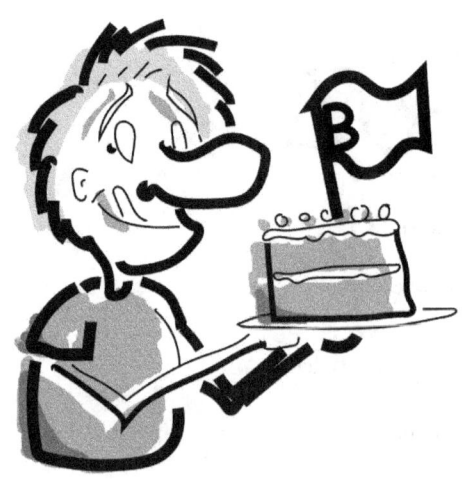

The Never-Ending Diet Rollercoaster

The diets to help you are endless!
Don't worry 'cause you'll never spend less!
You give them some money
For words just like honey
Sweet promises that are so generous

Most diets all come with prediction
To lose weight you must use restriction
You cut out some foods
While you mess with your moods
And you follow a whole lot of fiction!

Remember when you are restrictive
The quick fix becomes quite addictive
On each diet rebound
Some new weight will be found
This phenomenon is quite predictive

What to Eat?

But what does your poor body need?
Three vegies and meat, a good feed
Some fruit and some dairy
Here's nothing that's scary
Your energy needs don't exceed

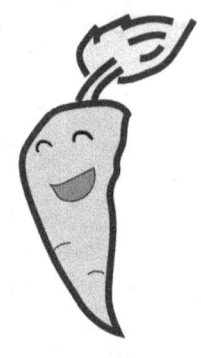

Don't cut out one food or another
Take heed to the words of your mother
Don't go the extreme
Just so you can be lean
Please don't look like your ten year old brother!

The body's simplistic complexion
Needs food from five groups for digestion
Like a well-oiled car
It will then go quite far
When you follow these rules of ingestion

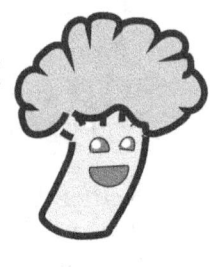

Some vegies and fruit are a must!
A good butcher is someone to trust
Some food from the cow
And a treat we allow
And a great loaf of bread with a crust

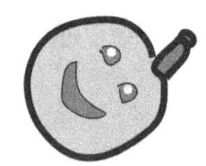

Your portions are then made quite fast
You must eat so your energy lasts
With your goals in your mind
Tip the balance you'll find
The results will be what you have asked!

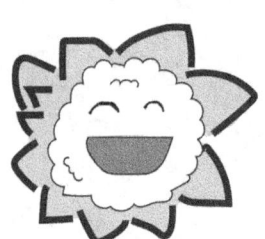

Beware ... The Lucrative World of Impression!

The lucrative world of impression
Has half the world in an obsession
You take and injection
To look like perfection (whose version?)
And end up with a health concession

Don't fall for the bull and the hype
You're perfect whatever the type
Please just be yourself
It is your own wealth
Like a flower or fruit that is ripe

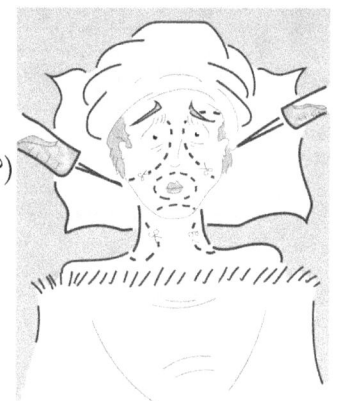

My Tip ...

Decide what you want from the start
What is good for your soul and your heart
Then you make a great plan
With support if you can
Write it down in a book or a chart

When you think of the food keep it straight
Use the rules of the two and the eight
Take eighty from ground
Then twenty is found
In the packets which man would create

When you look back in time you will see
That you create your own destiny
When you follow your plan
From the day you began
You will make yourself happy and free!

A Little Anatomy and Physiology

When I look at my body
I view with respect
I know I am something unique
The way that I move
The way that I look
Is something about which I shall speak

I know I can run
I know I can jump
I see myself moving about
When sprinting, I puff
Exertion's quite tough
A system, quite complex, no doubt

The parts of my body
They move in conjunction
I know after thinking a thought
That patterns evolve
From the young to the old
We all do what our body's been taught

Some parts of us though
Like our heart and our lungs
Act according to something internal
Unconscious commands
Fulfil life's demands
Our existence, our flame, quite external

The Musculo-Skeletal System
Provides us a framework to live
It is made of such parts
Like we see on those charts
A list of them now I will give

There are bones and there's muscles
Ligaments, joints
Some cartilage and tendon, a tether
Connective tissue
Important, we know
Supports and binds it all together

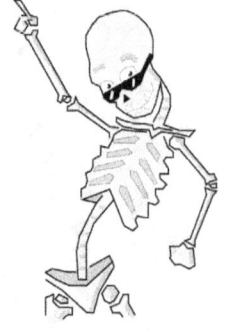

Without all these parts
What would we look like?
I think, just one great blob of jelly
No form, no support
All movement abort
No difference between arms or my belly

Apart from all this
I must not forget
Some other important functions
Protect and support
Your organs, your gut
And movement where bones reach a junction

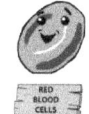

Producing blood cells
A number one thing
Without them you just cannot do
But wait there is more
In bones you will store
Some-phosphorus and calcium too

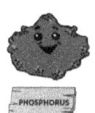

Thermostasis
A temperature gauge
Your muscles are playing this game
Whatever the set
In cold or in wet
You temperature will be the same

Last but not least
Aesthetics, they please
We all like a good-looking 'bod'
Well proportioned
Muscle definition
Is something which we all applaud!

The skeletal man
Divided in two
Has axial and appendicular
All the bits of your frame
See your chart for the name
Their categories are quite particular

continued...

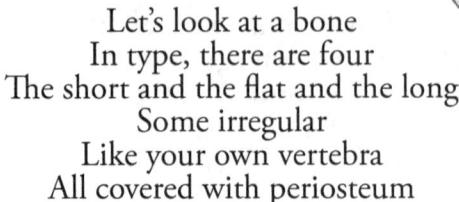

Let's look at a bone
In type, there are four
The short and the flat and the long
Some irregular
Like your own vertebra
All covered with periosteum

The number of bones
I see in a babe
We know is the sum of three hundred
Two hundred and six
With an x-ray take pics!
In a man or a woman are numbered

Let's look at a joint
It's how we all move
In type there are three that I know
Some move quite a lot
Some are fixed to a spot
And some little movement allow

The fibrous, your skull
The synovial
The hinge and the ball and the socket
Gliding, in your wrist
When you move and you twist
The radius and ulna will pivot

Let's not forget
The cartilaginous
Your vertebrae still like to move!
Bend forwards or back
On the field, on the track
On the dance floor now, see how we groove!

The number of muscles
We have in our frame
Is something that can be debated
From what I can see
Six hundred and forty
In type there are three that are rated

The voluntary
The ones we can move
Are found on the skeletal frame
They give us control
'To have and to hold'
Without them life would-not be the same

The smooth, in our gut
Aid digestion and blood
And the cardiac muscle's our heart
These are involuntary
They can't be contrary
Intrinsic to life and its part

One more thing I can see
When our movement is free
That our muscles can only contract
As one muscle releases
And the other decreases
It is then that you have your impact

An example we see
When you're bending your knee
The hamstrings will shorten, and pull
The quads on the top
Release, sort of flop
And your movement is strong and is full

They work like a clock
As they coordinate
One action, that comes from decision
Each time that you move
Please remember how you've
Got a marvellous organism

And so you will see
In their complexity
This system is really remarkable
I trust how it works
I enjoy all its perks
It gives me some joy and some sparkle

A Case of Intimidation!

The big, bold body
Bounces up to the barbell
And braces his back
Buttocks and biceps
He breathes and bares the
Bar on his back
As he bends his knees
He believes his body is the best
And puts it to the test
His squats are slow and steady
And his strength is
Exerted as he pushes upwards
He strains and steadies himself
Silently exhilarated at the
Success he sees
Each session strengthening
His muscles and sinews
Solid in his
Performance statistics!
He is resolved and purposeful
The power of his presence
Permeates the place
As onlookers peer
And silently praise
His performance
He is pleased
And punches the air
Persistence and perseverance
Are prevalent
And he pushes through
Semi-permanent barriers
And makes practical progress
On the pathway to success

Part Three ...
The Art of Being an Entrepreneur

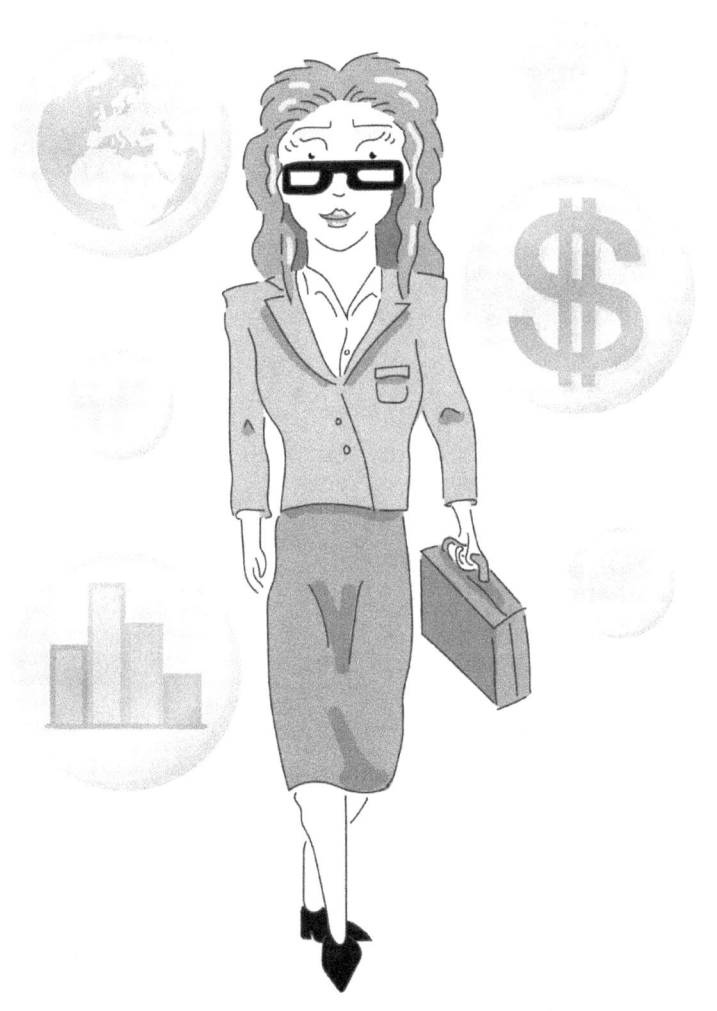

Les Mills ... International Glory

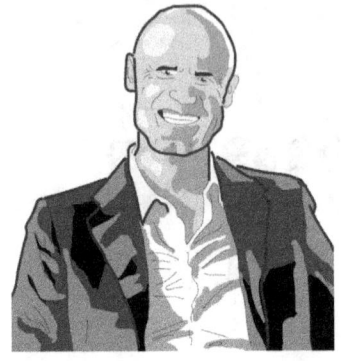

What was there before 'Les Mills'?
A vast, and empty void
A space and place not yet defined
No format yet employed

I try so hard to get a glimpse
Of worlds without these icons
It doesn't seem conceivable
In years that are bygone

When I look back I see his path
Determined by objective,
But what conceptual thought provoked
A movement, so effective?

Inside the heart of every man
Lies talent and emotion
To grow, create, design his life
From one small thought or notion

I know at all times, in my world
I'm thinking and creating
I see a need and then design
Solutions without waiting

It comes to me, as well, to you
Our need for growth and learning
"Expansion," cries the Universe
It's what you all are yearning

And though we sit and calculate
The pros and cons of matter
The present time cannot reveal
The former and the latter

I think when Phillip Mills designed
His product, many live by
He must have seen a flash of light
And thought, "I'll give this a try"

What makes a product like his great?
In logic I will reason
Follow structure and design
A plan for every season

Find a void, a lack, a need
Then work out a solution
Then tell the world how you can help
And start a revolution!

I'm sure that in the longest weeks
There was much doubt and fear
But lots of work, and time, and thought
Eradicates that sphere

Great businesses come by design
The pattern that they use
Is tried and tested by the bold
It is a path they choose

When you design something unique
The world will stand in awe
For people love to try what's new
It's what they're living for

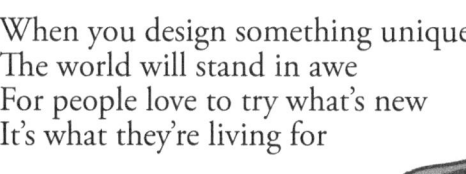

continued...

'Les Mills' has something quite unique
It benefits so many
The clubs and the participants
Have value for their penny

They have a structure, proven true
With room for much expansion
Something to suit 'most every one
An ever growing mansion

They make us fall in love with fit
They make the hard seem easy
They give us an experience
That will not leave us queasy

There's room for personality
Instructors add the flavour
They're trained to give the best they can
Their energy you'll savour

They play upon our need for love
The crowd and atmosphere
Looking good and working out
With friends and with our peers

So many things 'Les Mills' does well
Creating motivation
I know when I go to a class
I feel the stimulation

I'd hate to watch a football match
And be just one spectator
I'd rather be with lots of friends
Who are participators

Being part of something big
A sense that I belong
Connects me universally
I feel so safe and strong

***

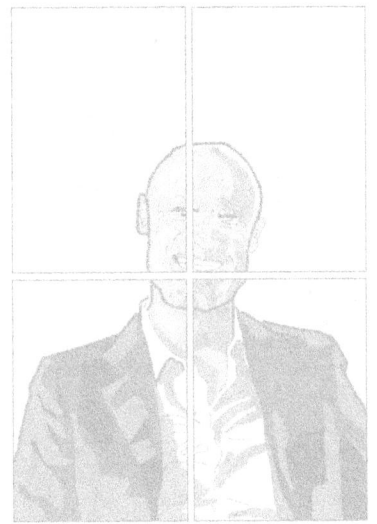

How global has the world become?
We are now one big nation
We have advanced beyond our realm
Each mark a generation

But though we're rich in many ways
We're seeing so much wealth
There's one thing right before our eyes
Concerning our poor health

The world has need to reconcile
We're so out of proportion
An epidemic fills the world
Creating a distortion

The lack of health, the rising tide
Of sickness and disease
Still holds us back, it keeps us low
It brings us to our knees

We've needed help in many ways
And 'Les Mills' takes the glory
The worldwide cry for help was heard
We now share his life's story

His dream was big, and now we see
A movement universal
So, thank you Phil, for your back yard
It was your dress rehearsal

The 'Les Mills' program that we know
Has helped the world immensely
Adherence to the principles
And structure held intensely

It is a light to all around
And we can see a measure
Some principles we can apply
To make our life a treasure

continued...

The reason for Phil's great success
Is obviously clear
He did something he loved to do
Something that he held dear

And when the program took to flight
He used no limitations
His product grew, fulfilled a need
Expanded to the nations

I wonder what we'll see ahead
On canvas is the story
I sense that everything will be
With honour and with glory

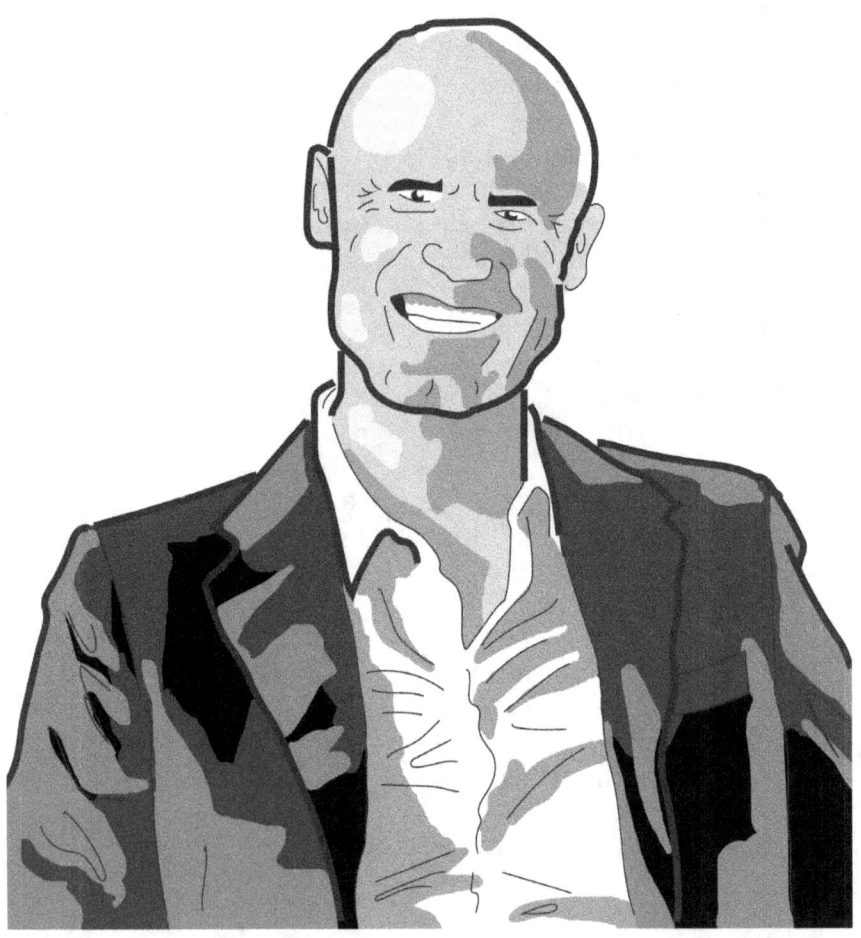

A Chat with Zig Ziggler

Last night I had a chat with Zig
I asked him his advice
He took a moment from his day
It was so very nice

I asked him for his number one
A message he would bring
He said that you should have a dream
In which you are the king

Your goals are so important, dear
They are the guiding light
Without them you're just wandering
Like blind men in the night

I see the world so full of men
I know with just a glance
They do not have a goal or dream
They do not have a chance

So take a moment of your time
These words I heard from Zig
To really know just want you want
Be bold, look far, dream big!

In every detail be exact
In planning use precision
Your target makes your path, my friend
Affecting each decision

To be effective they must cause
A consequence outstanding
They must require you to change
They must be quite demanding

They must be big, please specify
Your purpose and your meaning
And every day, in every way
Towards them you'll be leaning

The bigger picture helps you see
With focus and with clarity
The smaller tasks you do each day
Are done with no disparity

Build foundations for your life
By working and believing
And you will find eventually
Much fruit you are receiving

I pondered at the message
And at my life so far
I knew that I had done so much
I'd followed my north star

But, what to do this moment?
I took an inventory
I decided I must write
A new and different story

I'd taken a new pathway
My life had changed so much
I'd learned to love and laugh again
I'd felt an Angel's touch

I found I had so much to do
A new, exciting plan
Something that would benefit
The Universe and man

The words from Zig I knew were right
And so I took some paper
Wrote down a list of all my goals
I was now my life's shaper

I made a target and a plan
My focus was directive
But like a missile in the air
The compass is corrective

Zig told me how he learned to fly
He said sometimes you fall
But confidence will come with time
And soon you will stand tall

So take a leap, have faith and trust
Take chances, do exploring!
And you will find that sure enough
On wings you will be soaring

"The weather is the weather"
It's neither good nor bad
Your attitude is what counts most
It could be great or sad

So if you want to spend your life
In higher altitude
Look at yourself in the eye
And change you attitude

Another thing that Zig expounds
Control your conversation
Be the first to greet a man
Please, be the inspiration

Look for good in all around
In man and circumstance
Your mission is, in life, my friend
To learn and to advance

"You've gotta ask the question"
You have to question why
Never stop enquiring
The wherefore and whereby

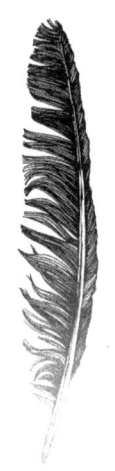

Don't take 'no' for an answer
Be resolute, unwavering
And every day you'll find that life
Towards you will be favouring

When walking through the paths of life
Keep focussed on your story
Don't fall for all the fallacies
With men and their own glory

"Don't let the turkeys get you down"
With vain talk and their gabbling
In other people's circumstance
Don't find yourself a dabbling

continued...

"Don't spend money you don't have"
The world has debt that's spiralling
Go and take a look at home
And see what goods are piling

Take a break from spending big
Use money that is yours
Save a bit, invest a bit
And give to some good cause

A few more words from this great man
Which give me inspiration
Are all around your heart and soul
And your own dedication

"Take time for you, please, just sit still"
Each day that you are living
In quiet contemplation
And a moment of thanksgiving

Take time for those who you love best
To them direct compassion
And with your time, which is a gift
Assign a needful ration

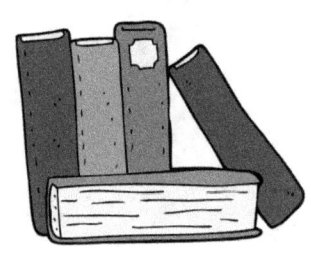

Your body too, needs love and care
To keep it strong and fit
Exercise and healthy food
Be prudent, wise, towards it

Zig tells us too about our mind
Don't fill it full of negatives
Put in there "the good, the clean
The powerful and positive"

"Read books about the greatest men"
With lives which you would sample
The ones whose words and deeds align
Who lead by their example

There's so much more that I could say
Zig's words could fill my pages
"Be supergood, flamboyant"
"Making monumental changes"

For you were born to fly, like
An aeroplane with wings
You were born for great success
So go, achieve great things

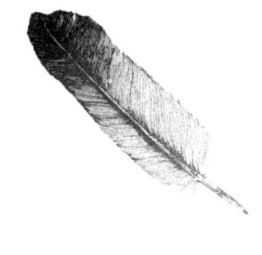

And in the act of stepping up
When all is said and done
What matters most is not the goal
It's what you have become

Stand tall and proud, please, do your best
Keep on your face a smile
The person that you have become
Does everything in style

I felt like I was talking to
A man, just like my dad
His good advice was full of love
Adventures he has had

I'm willing at this moment
To take his good advice
In all these things I'll do my best
You need not ask me twice

I'm focussed now, I have a list
Inside my heart and mind
To help me on my walk in life
My further purpose find

And though I'm turning fifty-one
There's so much more to learn
There's so much more for me to do
There's so much to discern

Success is something we become
How could we ever measure?
The 'something good' that we have done
Our life is our own treasure

In helping one, you help yourself
The art is in the giving
The picture that you paint of you
On canvas that is living

continued...

So, thank you, Mr Zig Ziggler
For being an example
A shining light to lead the way
A life that I could sample

And as a father to us all
We learn from men of glory
To be the star in our own show
The leader in our story

There's one more quote I'd like to add
It goes something like this
"Today is great and if you don't
Believe it, try to miss"

You miss just one, and then you'd know
How good it was to be!
There's something here for you to do
There's purpose here for me

So I can't wait for our next chat
I thank you for your words
When I think big, and look at me
It doesn't sound absurd

It's something that I now believe
I feel excitement rising
Accomplishments will come with ease
It will be quite surprising!

The Amazing... Walt Disney

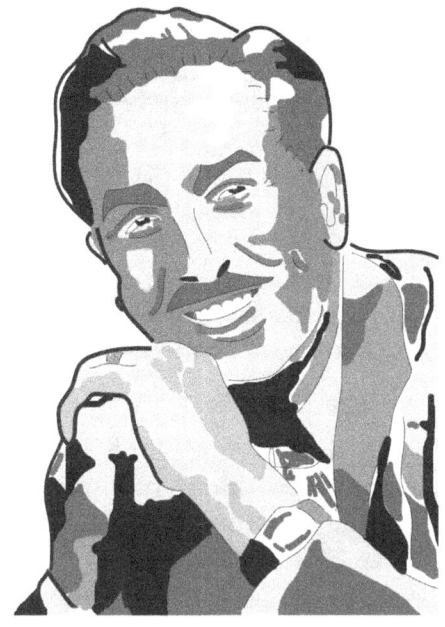

You can't stop a dreamer
You can't hold him down
He just wants to build and create
Don't tell him that something
Just cannot be done
To 'give up' he cannot relate

A man named Walt Disney
I view with respect
A man who's remembered by many
Started his life
By cartoon design
Was poor, without even a penny

He tried and he 'failed'
Some doors were slammed shut
He found himself knocked to the ground
A lesson just learned
He stood up once more
And was ready to 'play' the next round

continued...

He sat on a train
When all seemed to fail
Conditions, they really were sticky
Took out his pen
And started to draw
And came up with someone called Mickey

He drew and he planned
He never stopped thinking
Of all he could do and achieve
Took hold of ideas
And made them so real
In fantasies he did believe

With Roy by his side
Together they built
A company for entertainment
The spreading of wings
A little updraft
And soon there was just no containment

The Magical World
Of Disney would bring
Much joy to the lives of so many
A story book theme
Is one we all love
How could we deny this to any?

The vision expanded
And soon we would see
The fantasy had come to life
A Disneyland world
A place of retreat
Where most folks could forget their strife

To not settle back
When he had completion
Was something that Walter desired
And then at his death
The people would say
Walt Disney had never retired

His dreams were not finished
For that was his aim
Perpetual expansion of man
Guided through life
With godlike perception
Following a grandiose plan

He's one of a kind
Persistent, achieving
Stood firm when most others would fall
Believed in a dream
Created his life
From beginnings so humble and small

Some quotes from this man
Could help lift us all
We look to the entrepreneur
We all can be great
If we find our own path
And we would no longer defer

Keep moving ahead
And only look back
To see just how far you have come
Open new doors
Keep doing new things
Don't get lost in the pack or the scrum

Walt's life and his values
Were solid and firm
A structure that gave him great strength
When facing dilemmas
Or making a choice
Was able to keep at arm's length

The money was something
That gave to him choice
It wasn't his ultimate aim
Making more movies
Creating more fun
That was the name of his game

continued...

"I'd rather entertain
And hope people learn"
Walt Disney was quoted as saying
Than trying to teach
And then get a laugh
I'd rather see learning while playing

The nature of Walt
An inquiring mind
He always would question the why
If things didn't work
He'd look at the task
And think up some new way to try

He didn't relate
To critics at large
His focus remained firm and clear
He knew his desire
Was always to please
The audience that was so dear

A fairy tale life
One many would seek
Would see also trouble and pain
When times were quite bad
And all would seem lost
It is then there is so much to gain

The frailty of life
A gift to us all
The contrast within the great veil
Is something so firm
Yet also so weak
Inside we are both strong and frail

There lies within each
The young and the old
The lost and the lonely and sad
But also the child
With joy in the new
The fearless and the brave young lad

I'm looking at Walt
And in his example
I see how the mighty would fall
I see them rise up
From each trouble or strife
Rising up they would grow and stand tall

I see in their life
The values they hold
Integrity at the forefront
Great men are like gold
Are precious, a gem
Their challenges they would confront

Inside every man
There lies a great plan
Just waiting to flower and blossom
In every detail
Each individual
In their own way can be really awesome

So, 'never give up'
And 'never give up'
This quote is a cry to each man
Your purpose, dear friend
Go out and have fun
Be doing the best that you can

I thank you, dear Walt
For you touched my life
In touching the soul of the nation
A wheel in a wheel
Eternally turns
Successful without a completion

Keep looking at life
A way to grow up
In so many ways there are more
When one door swings shut
Another will open
Revealing a whole lot more

continued...

I look to those men
Who lead by example
Showing and leading the way
And take from their life
Such things as I need
To forge straight ahead on my way!

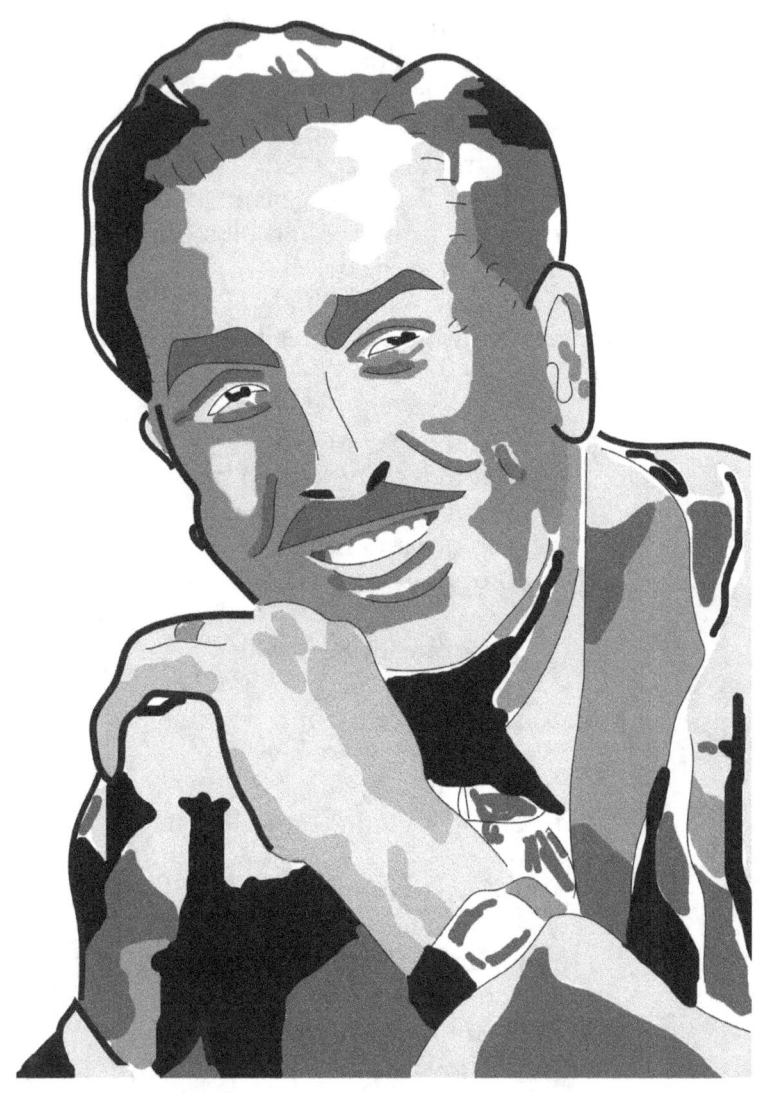

Why Do Businesses Fail?
And How to Make Yours a Success!

Why do businesses fail?
A question that needs some reviewing
People starting out in life
A business they're perusing
Would be advised to look ahead
To see what trouble's brewing
To see what things they can avoid
That could be their undoing

Number one on the list
Would be the question, 'Why?'
Are you doing what you love?
That causes you to fly?
Or are you offering some 'great'
Thing, that you won't even try
Selling something you don't love
Will leave you high and dry

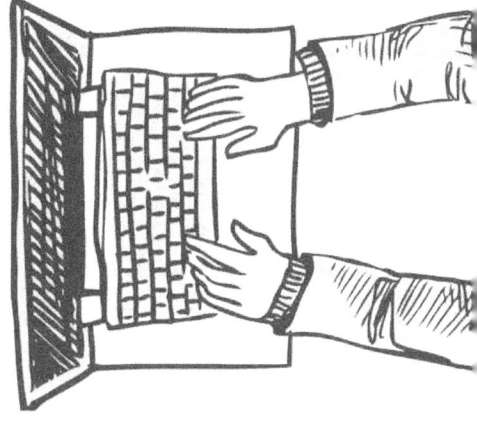

I think that the solution
For this one on the list
Is take an honest look inside
To see what train you've missed
You'd break your own dear heart
If you were to persist
Look at what you're doing
Your true purpose don't resist

Go and find another
A reason you must live
A passion that you have inside
A service you can give
For businesses that come from
Love, each moment will outlive
And you will find that in your soul
You will be positive

continued...

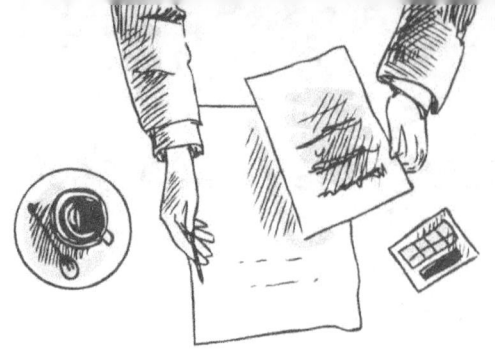

The next one we shall look at
Will be the question, 'What?'
What is it you're doing?
And what is it you're not?
Do you have the systems
That make an easy plot?
Or are you going round and round
All tied up in a knot?

Find a way that makes
The pathway smooth and slick
With systems that you have in place
Constructing brick by brick
Organising all things
Using every trick
Making all your processes
So easy and so quick

Obviously next
Will be the question, 'Where?'
Where did all the money go?
Who's sitting in that chair?
Do you have accounts,
Finances to compare?
Or has the money vanished
And gone up into 'thin air'

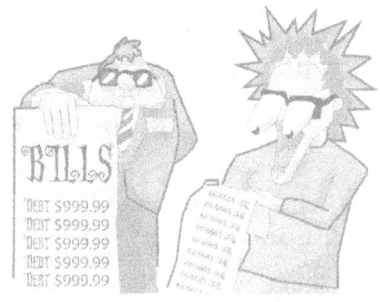

Overuse of credit
Buying too much stuff
Spending all your capital
When you just had enough
The bank is on your doorstep
Cause they see through your bluff
Now you're in big trouble
And the times are really tough

What you need to know
Is how to handle money
Use your common sense
Both when times are bad or sunny
Spending without planning
Will never end up funny
You must use your finances
Like bees around the honey

Plan and use it wisely
An inventory works
Then save a bit, invest a bit
Your future do not shirk
Pay yourself, your workers,
And each one of your clerks
And have a good accountant
Who will help you with the perks

Now we're getting closer
We're looking at the 'When?'
Do you have a plan
That you have written with a pen?
Something you can look at
To guide the 'now' to 'then'
How your business will succeed
Advice from some wise men

Did you think it through?
Or did you fail to plan?
Do you want to see your time
Go down the dunny can?
If you plan to fail
This project you began
Then just forget your common sense
Forget your business plan!

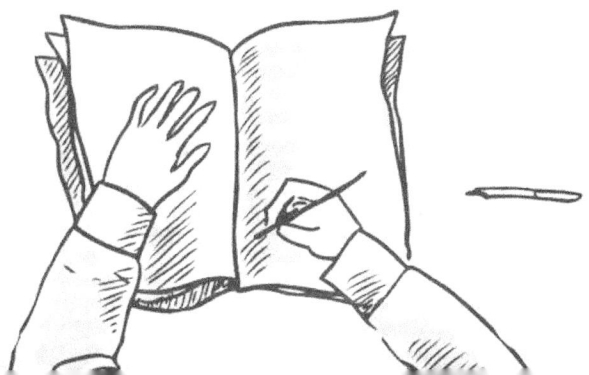

continued...

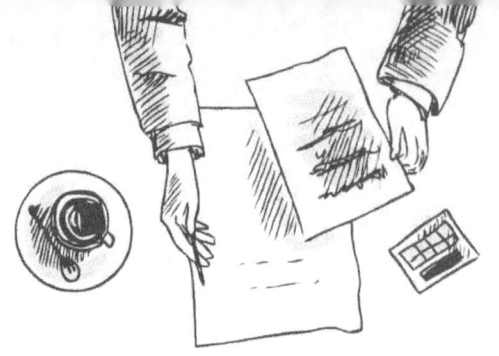

I know that's not your goal
I know that's not your mission
I know you have an awesome plan
I know you have good vision
I see you thinking through
With careful intuition
I see you taking good advice
I see you using wisdom

You plan has come to pass
Each detail is recorded
What you bought and purchased
Was what you had afforded
To each and every task
Sound knowledge was accorded
And all your efforts that you gave
Productively rewarded

You keep a detailed record
Of all you would achieve
You plan and use professionals
Their good advice receive
And then when you are dreaming
Of all you would conceive
You now know for certain
That is what you will receive

You're feeling pretty high
The hard work has been done
You've gracefully accomplished
All those things that you've begun
You followed good advice
Left nothing else undone
And as it has turned out
You found that it was awesome fun

How will you be feeling?
In this blessed state?
You would feel so fabulous
I barely can relate
I can feel your vibes
You're feeling really great
Life is just so splendid
Nothing else can quite equate

Give me your best words
I know you are excited
You did it! You're self-confident
You know you just can't fight it
Fantastic and impressive
Unstoppable, ecstatic
I'm proud of you, excited
You're an excellence fanatic!

You're extraordinary
A cut above the rest
In all things you're a champion
You love it! You're impressed!
How thrilled we are, it's awesome
And this amazing you
All because you took advice
And did what you could do

But hang on now, imagine
If all this was a lie
You didn't take our good advice
You are not flying high
You failed to do the homework
You failed to even try
And now you're sitting pondering
And asking yourself, why?

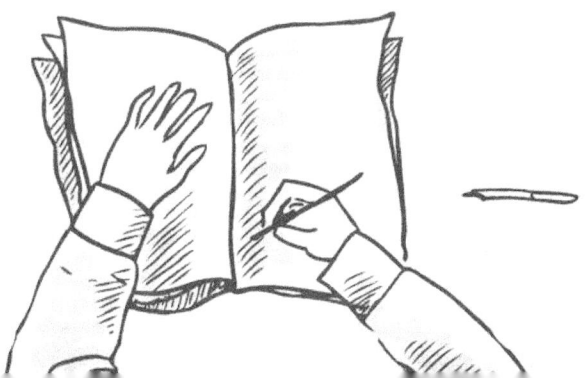

continued...

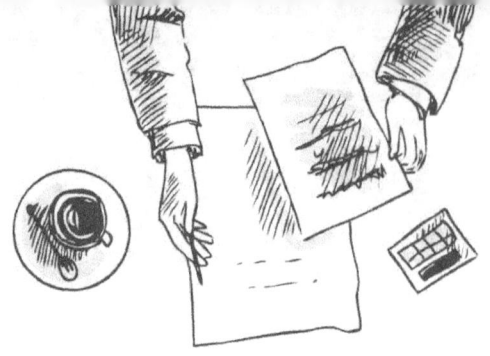

The road ahead is shrouded
With darkness all around
You've lost your sure footing
You're losing all your ground
You cannot pay the creditor
No money can be found
And you're afraid that they will come
Your life and soul impound

Your business is abysmal
You're feeling quite defeated
Life has been a struggle
And now you are feeling cheated
And all the people in the world
Can see you are defeated
All because you didn't take advice
Were you conceited?

How bad is all this trouble?
Your heart is in distress
Your business is a failure
And your life is quite a mess
There's no one in your life
That you could possibly impress
All because the fundamentals
You did not address

Give me your worst nightmare
The feelings are encrusted
A failure, a lie
Ashamed and so disgusted
You're sad and hypocritical
What was a golden hour
Has fallen with a mighty crash
Like some enormous tower

You're disappointed, sluggish
Depressed and quite deflated
So horrible and cranky
Every moment you're berated
What could be much worse
When looking in the mirror
You are unhappy with that man
Who's feeling so inferior

We're living in the moment
Today is all we get
It is where all decisions lie
Where challenges are met
If you do what you have done
What will your life beget?
Or do should you make a different path,
New goals and plans to set

Is there any help
That I could offer you?
I would say, 'Just be yourself
And follow what is true
Know your goals, your values
And make a good alliance
Use a little bit of sense
And quite a lot of science'

When you have a business
What do people see?
Do you have the sparkle?
The authenticity?
Are you doing something
That you would give for free?
And is it something we can have
In our reality?

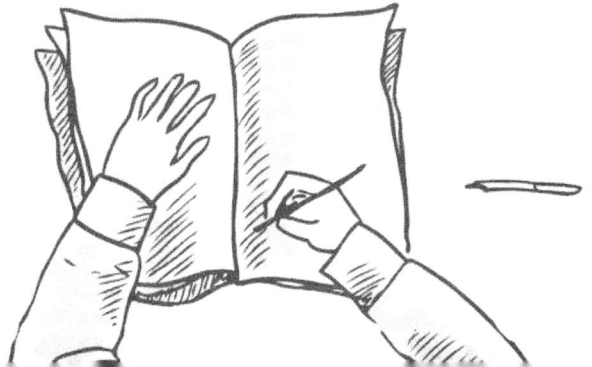

continued...

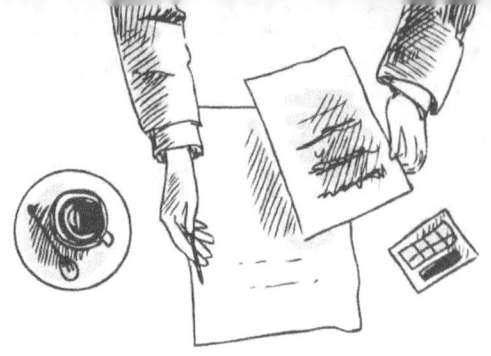

What are you prepared to do
To make you dreams come true?
Do you have the courage
And the strength to follow through?
Do you have commitment
For something that is new?
Do you make me feeling like saying
"Wow", when I leave you?

Is there still a fence?
A barrier so high?
That causes you to stay
Among the turkeys and not fly?
Is there still a problem
That you cannot deny?
Or can you rise up to the mark
And give a victory cry?

This moment we've created
Whatever we decide
Could take us up a mountain
Or some roller coaster ride
The choice is yours my friend
You can take it in your stride
Whatever action you take now
Could fill your heart with pride

I hope you choose a path
That will lead you to success
And not just leave it all to chance
And end up in a mess
I hope you take advice
Find yourself a mentor
And in your life you realise
That you are the inventor

For life is full of substance
Enough for everyone
Go outside and see the world
Be brave and have some fun!
Helping others on your way
A blessing to someone
Looking back then, you can say
That nothing was undone

If we had a program
To help you reach your mark
Would you now be interested?
To wisdom would you hark?
Can I show you something
That will give a bit of spark?
To help you get to sunshine
Be no longer in the dark?

The choice is yours my friend
I see you do perceive it
A gift from someone straight to you
I trust you will receive it
Just open up your hand right now
I know that you believe it
Whatever goal that you desire
I know you will achieve it!

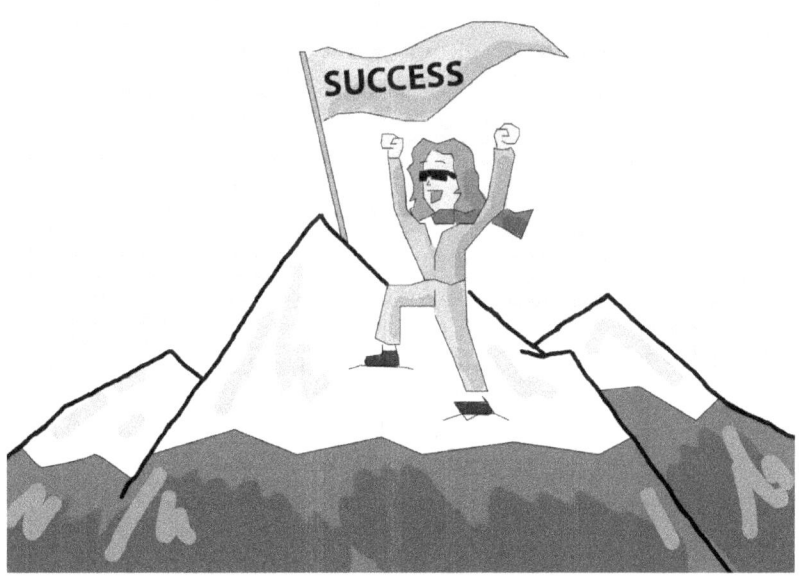

THE RISK...

You ask me about taking a risk?
Considering the odds
Making decisions with calculation
Pondering on futures
And possible outcomes
As I stand with my application
You give me facts and figures
Statistics and more
The pros and cons of choices
And you wonder
Is this a risk I should be taking?
Is this a decision I should be making?
To live?
To breathe?
To move forward
Into something
That may, or may not be successful?
May be quite stressful?
Something that requires me to grow?
Do you even know
How I got here?
Where it was I came from
And how I overcame
My fear?
Do you know what it's like
To stand against everything you've ever known
And walk out into the great unknown?
Not knowing if you would stand or fall
Moving to a place where you know nobody
At all
Where everything is new
And you feel so isolated
But you know the past
Is something that will never be
Recreated
Risk taking!
Future making!
Ground breaking!
Money making

Choices
I hear those voices!
And, in consideration
There is something I must say
Yes, I could walk alone
Go my own way
Start a new business
Decide my own pay
Going it alone has its perks, I know
But working with a team
Is quite another show
And this is what I'm choosing
If I choose to work with you
I'm purposefully launching out
Into something new
Doing something that I don't know
Will make me grow!
Expand myself
Learn new stuff
So what if the road
Is a little bit rough?
There is no problem
This is a fair call
You could be watching my success
Or you could see me fall
I can take the risk
This is who I am!
But I'm the one experimenting
With this future plan!
For the only form of failure
That I know
Is never even trying
Never giving it a go!

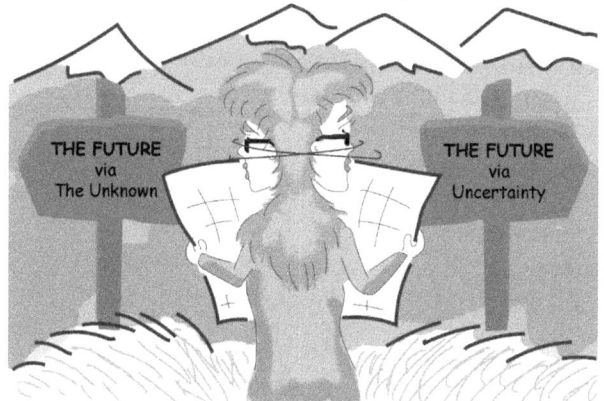

Who Am I?

Standing on the precipice of time
I find myself looking
At an overview
Of this life of mine

Visions of present, past and future
Merging into a kaleidoscope
Of thoughts, memories
And experiences

A journey beginning with one small step
Into something felt, seen, tasted
Touched and heard
But not yet understood . . .

As time rolls on, learning and growing
Teach us about who we really are
We discover
An inward knowing

Something intangible, yet so very real
The picture on canvas
Depicting the essence
Of the individual seal

The stamp of who I am is now recorded in history
By the footprints I leave in the sand
Sometimes unwittingly
And at other times, planned

The kaleidoscope changes
With the turning of the wheel
And I gain another perspective
Another way to feel

Always changing and reforming who I am
Today I am this person
Tomorrow. . .
Another man

Who Do I Believe In?

Who do I believe in?
I believe in me
I have found a lot of joy
In self-discovery

Looking at examples
Men who now stand tall
Facing much adversity
Rising up from fall

I am now my tower
See my inner strength
Standing up for who I am
Midst trials of great length

Who could see this future
Through the gloomy haze?
Who could see the path ahead
Inside this giant maze?

When I rose above it
Took a higher view
That was when the old life
Stepped out and I was new

An Angel's word of comfort
I see it now in part
Descended like a gentle dove
To mend my broken heart

A word, so fitly spoken
From many on my way
Was there to help this troubled soul
And guide me through my day

I thank those souls each moment
I send my gift of love
To each and every one of them
On earth and those above

A Vote of Thanks

I'd like to take a moment
To mention but a few
My husband, John became transformed
His soul he did renew

He could no longer live
That dark demeaning creature
Reformed himself in one great move
Now love and light's his feature

And we now have each other
We are no longer two
What was two paths, has now been joined
By love that's deep and true

We'll journey on together
We'll make this a joint venture
We'll do whatever WE decide
A life of great adventure!

Jo
What can I say about you, Jo?
My youngest child
Loving and so generous
And yet, a little wild

Your nature and your courage
Is something, unique and beautiful
You left a place that kept you bound
And oh, so very dutiful

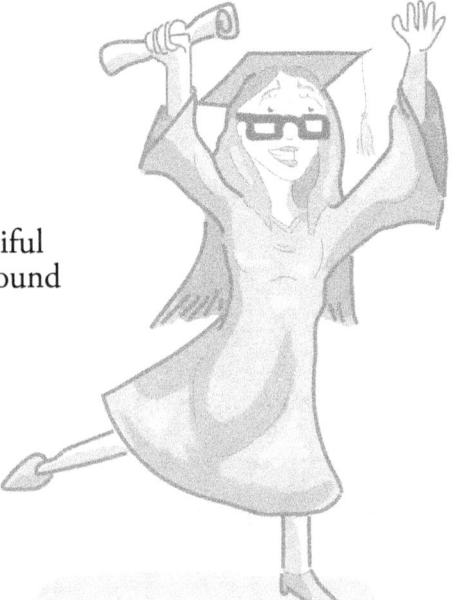

The frowns and glares of others
And here you are beside me
I am proud to be your mother

I see the path ahead for you
Is one of creativity
Getting back to nature
Finding your naivety

Connecting with the universe
This is your employment
And doing what you love to do
Will give you great enjoyment

Tom

For Tom, my friend and trainer
My life was saved by yours
The gift you gave, of who you are
Helped me to know my cause

I thank you for your guidance
Your common sense and logic
Was like a balm to heal my soul
Each training session magic

And though we trained the body
There was no separation
My mind and spirit grew as well
It was a preparation

And when the hour came
For death or for survival
I felt your touch upon my soul
And chose to see revival

I took a leap of faith
Looked back to all that growing
I found that deep within my heart
I had an inner knowing

An 'Angel sent to help me', Tom,
You are my inspiration
I now have strength within myself
You see my transformation

Max

To Kman and to Rowie
To Steve and all the crew
I offer my sincerest love
And say a big 'THANK YOU'

You made me look inside myself
And take a better view
You've helped me find a purpose
And live, for me, what's true

I saw in you a vision
Reflections of myself
A life that I could now create
A life with so much wealth

I left behind the darkness
The misery and hate
Decided I must claim my soul
Before it was too late

I listened to your wisdom
And took your good advice
I did those things required of me
No man need ask me twice

To find my own true purpose
With passion and sincerity
Has brought great joy and peace to me
A life of great prosperity

When I think about the future
I know for certainty
It's not so much 'bout what I'll do
But who I choose to be

Will I be true to who I am?
Compassionate, unique
Creative, inspirational
Determined now to speak?

Courageous as I look ahead
At what the future holds
Going forward, step by step
So positive and bold

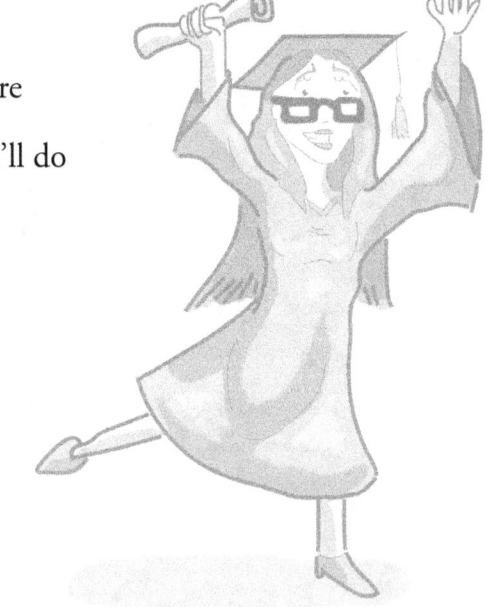

It took a while, dear Rowie
To figure some things out
Last night success was so far off
Today I sing and shout

Steve, I value your message
And your teaching
And when for new goals and visions
I am reaching

I will always look first
AT WHO I AM
And use those values
To figure out the next plan . . .

Kman, the game of life for me
Will first involve
Where I place my feet
And how I revolve

Moving my body in a dance like motion
Like the waves and the toss of the ocean
Defending myself from attack
Learning when to strike

And when to hold back
Being prepared and standing my ground
Never a moment unguarded be found
Taking advice that is true and is sound

And getting up, when I fall down
And being a winner
By playing my best game
Linda Skerman

That is my name
Proud to be me
And I'll never be the same
As yesterday, because today . . .

I am free!

My mountain has a climax
The hard work has been done
When one door closes, sure enough
There'll be another one

I know for me life holds a dream
Involving so much fun
I plan to live, and love and laugh
My goal ... To reach the sun!

The "Max Empowerment Program"
If I may call it that
Can be a platform for success
If change is where you're at

A step by step example
Of men who have a mission
Whose goal in life is helping those
Who want a clearer vision

With eyes to see a future
That you could now create
Begin, my friends, refine yourself
Please, do not hesitate

And if you need assistance
Look to your left and right
You may find help, like my 'MAX' friends
To help you through your night

Supporting my endeavours
I see these friends of mine
I saw them all along my way
Now at this finish line

And so it stands, I'm proud of us
At this, our graduation
We stand today for what we've done
LET'S ROCK this celebration!

Start from the heart

Discover your why

Cast off the fear

And then, my friend

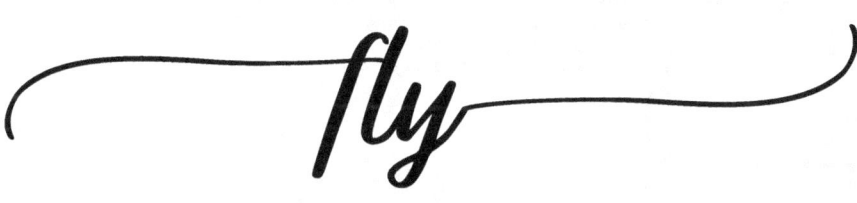

About the Author

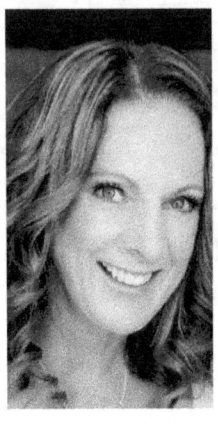

Linda Skerman is a prolific poet and writer who has taken her life to the written word in an extraordinary kaleidoscope of imagery and adventure, capturing major events that have changed her world and shaped her life relationships.

Linda is a gentle, life loving soul, married with four adult children and six grandchildren. She has lived in Queensland (Toowoomba) for most of her married life, and is now settled in Sandgate/Brighton in North Brisbane for the next chapter of her life which has only just begun.

She has been many things to many people, apart from wife and mother, a nurse, gymnastics coach, piano teacher, Personal Trainer, Jazzercise instructor and qualified Kinesiologist.

Her poetry has been shared in Brisbane and South East Queensland at poetry slams, open mics and speed poet events. She also won the prestigious walk-in poets award at the Woodford Folk Festival in 2017. An amazing feat in her own creativity, was having all Certificate IV in Fitness assignments and Diploma of Fitness Business assessment pieces completed and submitted as poetry, something that set her apart to graduate as Student of the Year, gaining the respect of trainers and fellow students.

Linda has followed many genres in poetry and writing, including physical training and diet, humour and many reflective pieces describing her personal experiences of her life journey and the world around her. Linda's deep sensitivity allows her to capture the essence of the portrait from many perspectives.

Her poetry for this entertaining and selectively insightful work is from the heart, touching and embellishing experience, learning and the life culture that is physical fitness.

Connect with Linda at:
www.facebook.com/insightstrengthtrainingforwomen
www.facebook.com/rippleinthepondpoetry
lindaskerman.author@gmail.com

www.ingramcontent.com/pod-product-compliance
Lightning Source LLC
Chambersburg PA
CBHW072103290426
44110CB00014B/1802

www.ingramcontent.com/pod-product-compliance
Lightning Source LLC
Chambersburg PA
CBHW042053290426
44110CB00006B/174